Chinese Herbs in the Western Clinic
A Guide to Prepared Herbal Formulas
Indexed by Western Disorders
& Supported by Case Studies

by Andrew Gaeddert, Herbalist

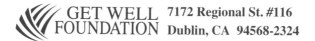

GET WELL FOUNDATION
7172 Regional St. #116
Dublin, CA 94568-2324

Disclaimer

This book is intended as a reference for practitioners. It should not be used as the sole basis for evaluating and treating patients. Non-practitioner readers should consult with their health care provider about suggestions made in this book, and before any suggestions are administered. Pregnant or lactating women should be administered herbs only under the direction of an experienced health care provider.

Chinese Herbs in the Western Clinic

Published by:
Get Well Foundation
7172 Regional St. #116
Dublin, CA 94568-2324

Distributed by:
North Atlantic Books
P.O. Box 12327
Berkeley, CA 94701

Production and typography by Bergner Communications
Copyediting by Eileen Ridge
Cover design by Cornerstone Graphics

Chinese Herbs in the Western Clinic is published by Get Well Foundation, a non-profit organization whose purpose is to educate the public and health care providers about natural therapies that are complements to Western medicine. Publications, symposia, and community-based research projects are planned.

ISBN 0-9638285-0-9 : $15.95

HOW TO ORDER

Single copies may be ordered from Get Well Foundation, 7172 Regional St. #116, Dublin, CA 94568-2324.

For trade, bookstore, and wholesale inquiries, contact North Atlantic Books, P.O. Box 12327, Berkeley, CA 94701.

Acknowledgements

I'd like to thank my parents LouAnn and Orlan Gaeddert for their suggestions, Carol Eckels and Patricia Puckett for their encouragement, and Jean Benge for her help in bringing this project to fruition.

.

Table of Contents

Foreword

Medical herbalism differs from folk herbalism in that medical herbalism is practiced in the context of a medical diagnosis, is used for the full range of conditions that afflict humanity, and its practitioners depend for their livelihood on obtaining good results. The three living systems of medical herbalism in the U.S. are the naturopathic tradition, the British tradition, and traditional Chinese medicine. Of the three, Chinese herbalism is by far the most developed. It has been continuously refined over thousands of years, to the point that it is now more sophisticated in its clinical applications than the pharmacy of Western biomedicine. By this I mean that indications, contraindications, and potential side effects are better known in the Chinese system, and that formulations are devised to minimize side effects that would be considered a tolerable nuisance in the Western system. Furthermore, Chinese medicine can treat many conditions for which Western medicine has nothing to offer—most notably the deficiency syndromes treated with Chinese tonic herbs.

The minimization of side effects while maintaining clinical efficacy is the chief benefit of Chinese formulas to the Western clinician. When side effects to Chinese formulas occur, they tend to be minor. This compares with 6-10% of hospital admissions in the U.S. due to adverse drug reactions — more people die in this country each year from adverse drug reactions than are killed in traffic accidents. The problems do not arise only with the strong drugs used in life-threatening situations. A large percentage of serious injury and death comes from gastrointestinal bleeding or kidney damage from simple pain medications. Chinese medicine has effective herbal treatments for pain, some of the included in this book, that have no such risky side effects.

The greatest obstacle for the Western practitioner in applying Chinese herbal formulas is the different diagnostic system in Chinese medicine. *Chinese Herbs in the Western Clinic* helps to bridge the gap between the two systems by categorizing formulas first by Western condition, and then differentiating among appropriate formulas for that condition according to Chinese principles. The book also includes extensive materials to introduce the Western practitioner to Chinese medicine.

i

Formulas in Chinese herbalism range from the personalized herbal formula, usually a tailored adaptation of a classical formula, to the *patent* or *prepared* formula, a mass-produced form used throughout China and Southeast Asia by practitioners and consumers alike. Because of the different climate, diet, and lifestyle in the U.S., prepared formulas from Asia cannot simply be prescribed by rote. Over the last few decades, appropriate modifications of Chinese prepared formulas have been made with Westerners in mind. The applications of these modified formulas, most of them now produced in North America, are what Mr. Gaeddert offers us in *Chinese Herbs in the Western Clinic.*

Paul Bergner
Editor
Medical Herbalism
February 1994

Notes on special terminology

Traditional Chinese Medicine (TCM) is based on an entirely different philosophical framework than Western biomedicine. TCM assumes that the individual is more than just the body; subtle properties such as "Heat," "Cold," "Qi" (energy), "Yang" (active principle) or "Yin" (receptive principle) are basic to TCM. Furthermore, TCM assumes a unity between the physical and the psycho-spiritual; thus terms in TCM such as "Heart" include the physical heart, but also include the conscious mind and the spirit. Throughout this book, to distinguish TCM terminology from corresponding Western terms, we capitalize the Chinese term. Thus the word Liver will mean the Chinese term, which includes the physical liver as well as the regulation of the flow of emotions; liver, on the other hand, is the Western term, and means the physical liver only. Those unfamiliar with any terms encountered may consult the glossary in the back of the book. Those unfamiliar with TCM may want to learn more by reading additional books or by attending classes or seminars to fully appreciate the philosophical framework of TCM.

Throughout the book, standard dosage frequencies are abbreviated as follows:

BID	two times daily
TID	three times daily
QID	four times daily

To the Practitioner

This book is designed as a reference guide for practitioners who use prepared formulas (tablets and capsules) primarily or as a follow-up or alternative to individually-tailored decoctions. Prepared formulas can yield surprisingly good results, but selection of the correct formula is essential. Those unfamiliar with herbs should consult practitioner manuals such as the *Health Concerns Clinical Manual* or the *K'an Herbal Formulas Guide*, which explain the patterns addressed by each particular formula in detail. For practitioners without extensive training in herbs, it remains important to work with an experienced herbalist for difficult cases or for cases that don't respond to prepared formulas.

Practitioners who combine acupuncture and herbal medicine almost always get better results than their colleagues who exclusively use acupuncture. This is because some conditions respond much better to herbal therapy than to acupuncture. However, acupuncture provides the valuable service of relaxing the patient. In the case of pain relief, acupuncture is more effective than herbal medicine but herbs help patients sustain treatments between acupuncture appointments. Finally, because of the bombardment of stress, poor diet, and excessive lifestyle that most Americans are exposed to, and the poor condition most patients are in by the time they see a practitioner, these patients need all the help they can get. Hopefully, this book will give an appreciation of the beauty of differential diagnosis (the heart of Chinese medicine) and will inspire further study.

This book will show you how to suggest a formula that takes into account the Western diagnosis, and suggests prepared formulas that have been successfully used for the particular condition, keeping in mind that the Western disease may be differentiated into several Chinese medical syndromes.

Three important syndromes for beginners

For the beginner in Chinese herbal medicine, the most important energetic properties to be familiar with are Excess Heat, Excess Cold, and Excess Dampness (see Major Energetic Imbalances). It is also important to differentiate between chronic and acute conditions. Keeping these factors in mind will greatly assist in the prescribing of Chinese herbal formulas.

I believe it is possible to achieve the 80-90% success rate using herbs by becoming familiar with these three imbalances. This does not mean their Western disease is cured; it means that the patients begin to feel better and their overall quality of life is improved.

For simple cases such as cold or flu, patients can start feeling better a couple of hours after taking herbs, depending upon the practitioner's ability to give the appropriate therapy at the right time. Even if one merely understands the three energetic imbalances, results can usually be seen within twenty-four hours. Of course chronic conditions take longer, but herbal treatment can still yield good results when taking these patterns into account when prescribing.

Formulation in Chinese medicine

The strength of Chinese herbal medicine is the concept of balance. Herbs are used in combination to strengthen effects of some herbs and eliminate any undesired effects of others. Some Chinese herbs are available in single herb form, but taking them this way greatly increases the chances of a negative reaction. It also ignores the beauty of Chinese medicine, which prescribes herbs according to syndrome differentiation. Some Western research has been conducted on Chinese herbs and formulas, but the most important aspects of herbs and formulas are their energetic properties and how these interact with the energetic properties of the patient.

For Westerners, an important category of Chinese herbs is the tonics, which are usually included in formulas. There is nothing like them in allopathic or homeopathic medicine. Tonic herbs will strengthen resistance to disease, and help the patients improve their overall health and feelings of well-being. If prescribed with the above categories in mind, these tonics can be taken safely for long periods of time by those who are under a lot of stress, or by those who are not in good health.

Usually a formula for long-term administration will contain some tonics and some herbs to treat specific symptoms, and other herbs that will help the body utilize the tonic herbs. Tonic herbs taken by themselves are too difficult to digest for most people, while herbs that relieve specific symptoms may actually drain the body's energy; that is why they work so well in conjunction with tonics, which help to replenish energy.

A modern formula

Let's look at a modern formula, Astra Isatis. This formula contains an extract of two antiviral and antibacterial herbs: Isatis leaf (Da Qing Ye), and Isatis root (Ban Lan Gen). These herbs are included to attack virus or bacteria. Astragalus (Huang Qi) and Codonopsis (Dang Shen) are two tonic herbs in this formula that enhance the immune system, according to modern scientific reports. More important, these herbs are warm energetically and help balance the Cold properties of the Isatis and Laminaria (Kun Bu). The latter is included because it reduces lymphatic swelling, which is associated with viral activity. Bupluerum (Chai Hu) is an interesting herb which helps to improve the liver function, and has been used as an ingredient in hepatitis formulas for thousands of years, long before Westerners learned to diagnose hepatitis. Epimedium (Yin Yang Huo) is used to replenish the Kidney energy, which is important to the function of the overall health of the body according to traditional Chinese medicine. Lycium (Gou Qi Zi) treats aching back and legs, promotes the regeneration of liver cells, and lowers blood cholesterol. Additional herbs help support the digestive system, and also help balance the formula so that it does not cause Excess Cold or Excess Heat (Cold or Hot syndromes).

An ancient formula

An example of an ancient formula is the Eight Treasure Formula (Ba Zhen Tang). This formula is for Blood and Qi deficiency in TCM. Its Western applications are anemia, irregular menstruation, and postmenstrual fatigue. This formula contains the well-known blood builder Tang-kuei, along with other blood builders such as Red Dates (Da Zao). Equally important are Qi tonics such as Ginseng or Codonopsis (Dang Shen), since the ancient saying is "without Qi, Blood cannot be built effectively." From a Western standpoint many of these Qi tonics improve both the immune system and the digestive system. It is interesting to note that a Chinese herbal formula for building the blood contains only a few blood tonics; the rest of the herbs are to help the body utilize the blood tonics. Herbs that help digest the blood tonics include Ginger (Gan Jiang) and Baked Licorice (Zhi Gan Cao); herbs such as Peony (Bai Shao), and Ligusticum (Chuan Xiong) help circulate the Blood tonics.

Modern and ancient combined

Stomach Tabs is a modern formula based on the ancient formula Ping Wei San. Several herbs such as magnolia (Hou Po), Citrus (Chen Pi) help improve digestive function, whereas pinellia (Ban Xia) helps reduce Phlegm, which according to TCM causes symptoms such as diarrhea. Bupleurum (Chai Hu) is a modern addition to this formula, since this herb is stress-reducing according to modern scientific experiments. According to both Chinese and Western medicine, stress can cause digestive upset and is a main causative factor in Irritable Bowel Syndrome (IBS). According to TCM, the etiology of most digestive disorders is Liver-invades-the-Stomach/Spleen, thus the addition of Bupleurum helps keep the Liver energy from attacking the Stomach. Oryza (Guya) is a modern addition to correct food accumulation. Many people in the West suffer from food accumulation, simply because we overeat and also tend to stuff our bodies with greasy foods that just sit in the stomach.

We have listed an example of a modern Chinese herbal formula, an ancient formula, and a modern formula developed from an ancient formula. The reader will surely appreciate that Chinese herbal formulas are far more than one active ingredient with some fillers added.

Major Energetic Imbalances

Cold pattern

A person with several of these symptoms predominant is considered to have a Cold pattern, and should be treated accordingly.

Cold hands and feet (can also be due to Liver pattern)
Cold back
Low energy
No desire
Fearful
Frequent urination
Pale tongue
Feel better in the summer
Rarely sweat
Employed outdoors
Loose stools
Weak voice
No desire to drink
Clear or white phlegm
Lack of appetite
Clear urine
Dizziness
Edema

Constitutional formulas

Spleen tonics such as Astra 8 or Kidney tonics such as Backbone are good. You may include one tablet of Quiet Digestion with each dose if there are any digestive problems. Power Mushrooms may be taken in addition, one or two tablets TID. Start slowly and build up to the full dose.

Additional considerations

Those who have a Cold pattern frequently feel cold all over. Korean or Chinese Ginseng is warming, as is fresh ginger cut up into thin slices as tea. Moderate lean meat, moderate spices, and moderate alcohol (one or two glasses wine per day) may be recommended. Walnuts and scallions are good. Eliminate all cold and raw foods, except fresh fruit. Discontinue fruit juices. Try to start exercising on a regular basis.

Hot pattern

A person with several of these symptoms predominant is considered to have a Hot pattern, and should be treated accordingly.

Feel warm all over
Frequently thirsty
Take medication, smoke
Feel stress, anxiety
Insomnia
Constipation
Red tongue
Athlete
Feel better in winter
Sweat a lot
Afternoon slump
Dark urine
Loud voice
Dominating, aggressive
Easily upset
Overly-emotional
Dry cough
Yellow phlegm or sputum
Irritable
Thin
Early and heavy menstruation, bright red blood
Easily angered

Constitutional formulas

Yin tonics such as Calm Spirit, Nine Flavor Tea and Wise Judge are appropriate.

Additional considerations

Those with a Hot pattern tend to feel hot and become agitated easily. American Ginseng is appropriate, but avoid Korean and Chinese Ginseng. For stress, use Calm Spirit, one to three tablets TID, and Ease 2 (with loose stools) or Ease Plus (with normal stools or constipation), one to three tablets TID. Wise Judge is especially good with a dry throat. Emphasize cooked vegetables and fresh fruit. In the summer raw vegetables may be okay. Fruit juices only occasionally, lean meat in moderation (2 oz. a few times a week). Eliminate dairy products, avoid alcohol, greasy or fried food, coffee. Avoid spicy foods, smoking. Try to avoid stress and strong emotions. Green tea is good, also Chrysanthemum tea. Try to meditate and relax as much as possible.

Damp pattern

A person with several of these symptoms predominant is considered to have a Damp pattern, and should be treated accordingly. A person with a Damp pattern may also have a simultaneous Cold or Hot pattern.

Indigestion
Food allergies
Heavy, overweight, bloated
Gas
Low energy
Moist tongue
Feel full/uncomfortable after eating (particularly yeast-containing foods)
Hard time at change of seasons
Hayfever
Sadness or depression (something weighing you down)
Catch the flu easily
Chronic disease
Helper personality
Office worker
Worry
Overweight
Live in a damp climate
Feel stuck
Greasy skin
Live or work in moldy place
Dull feeling
Dizziness

Constitutional formulas

Quiet Digestion is taken for several weeks to clear out the Damp-ness. Follow up with herbal formulas such as Six Gentlemen for Cold Damp conditions; for Damp Heat conditions such as candidiasis, use Phellostatin.

Additional considerations

Those with a Damp pattern frequently have digestive disorders and can feel as though they are covered by a wet blanket. Exercise that involves the stomach, such as situps, are good, but don't exercise to exhaustion. Acidophilus is good. Drink teas, especially peppermint, as this improves digestion. Avoid raw food, spicy food, alcohol, sweets, worry, sitting too much. Emphasize cooked vegetables, grains; avoid fruit juices, dairy products.

Chinese Herbal Preparations

Many American practitioners assume that the only traditional way of preparing Chinese herbs is by decoction, yet this is not true. According to Xu Dachun, the great 18th century Chinese physician: "Decoctions move fast. Their substance is light; their strength quickly subsides and does not stay. The effects of decoctions are especially fast when it comes to illnesses affecting the constructive or protective influences, the intestines and the stomach. In case of all other illnesses, either pills, powders or pastes may be appropriate."*

Only about 30 percent of the prescriptions found in the *Wushier Bing Fang*, a formulary dating from 168 BC China, are decoctions. It was common in China to administer formulas in powder, such as the famous Xiao Yao San. ("San" at the end of a formula means powder, whereas "tang" means decoction.) It was also a common practice to make pills by hand. These pills were rolled and mixed with honey.

Each method of administering herbs has its advantages and disadvantages. Thus, practitioners can choose not only the most appropriate formula for their patients, but also the most effective way to administer the herbs.

As our introductory quote suggests, even in China there is a long history of debate about the proper manner for prescribing and taking herbs. Much of the training given to students at American acupuncture schools is in prescribing herbal formulas for decoction. This overlooks a rich history in China of prescribing herbs in either pill, powder, paste, or tincture form. A comparison of teas, tablets, and tinctures will help practitioners have a better understanding of herbal delivery mechanisms. Teas for decoction, because they are composed of individual herbs, allow for a perfect match with the changing condition of the patient. This advantage has severe limitations, however, for the practitioner must have access to a well-stocked and maintained raw herb pharmacy. It is also difficult and time-consuming to learn this art of prescribing to practice it safely and effectively, not to mention the time required to fill raw herb formulas for patients.

Many practitioners feel that by brewing herbal teas, patients are more involved in their therapies. However, the American public does not share the Chinese cultural history of brewing and drinking herbal medicinal teas. Patient compliance is reduced because of the time and mess of brewing the herbs. Most of the formulas have an objectionable taste that many patients do not tolerate. Additionally, dosage levels fluctuate widely, since some patients either over- or under-cook their herbs, or boil off volatile oils by forgetting to cover the pot.

In contrast to teas, herbal tablets are taken easily at anytime, they have no objectionable taste, and provide accurate, consistent, controllable dosage levels. Most of the medicinal supplements taken are in pill form, partly because of their convenience. Tableted herbs assure higher patient compliance because Americans are accustomed to receiving their medicines in this form. Dr. Jianfu Jiang, professor at Emperor's College in Los Angeles suggests, "Tablets are suitable for treating long-term, chronic conditions where the patient must take herbs over a period time. Teas are especially useful for treating acute conditions."

In China, teas are commonly prescribed during the acute phase of an illness followed by pills during the chronic phase. One of the drawbacks of tableted herbs is that they are fixed formulas and are difficult to modify. One solution is to supplement a fixed, tableted formula with a modifiable tea. A brewed tea may be taken in the morning and at night, and tablets during the day. With this procedure the key is to determine which of the herbs are most suitable for powdering directly or for decocting and concentrating before pressing into tablets. Usually, as in the case of Ma Huang, above-ground parts respond best to concentrating. So above-ground herbs may be concentrated and added into tablets. Roots such as Astragalus and Ginseng are best powdered before tableting.

A large percentage of the practice of most clinicians consists of patients with chronic conditions. Teas and tinctures are useful for these cases, especially at the outset. However, over the long term, tablets are the best because of their convenience, higher patient compliance, and sustained dosage. It should be noted that it often takes three to four weeks before a tableted formula will show positive results in many chronic conditions at a normal dosage. A higher dose — even double or triple — can yield faster results.

Another form of herbs that is gaining popularity is the herbal tincture, because of its low manufacturing costs. Tinctures have a long history in China with traditional use reserved for Blood-activating formulas. Because alcohol enhances the delivery of medicinal effects to the musculoskeletal system, the alcohol format provides rapid uptake and quick results. For most other formulas tableting is preferable because it provides higher dosage levels and highest absorption at the lowest cost.

The disadvantage of tinctures is that the alcohol precludes their use by many patients. Because of its warming nature, alcohol is contraindicated in many Heat conditions, including Yin deficiency and excess Heat patterns. For example, alcohol could exacerbate Crohn's and other inflammatory conditions. Tinctures may also be inappropriate for recovering alcoholics or the alcohol-sensitive. Some practitioners recommend that the tinctures be placed in hot water to evaporate the alcohol before ingestion. But this procedure further dilutes a product that is already quite dilute, making it questionable if the dosage will be adequate at reasonable cost to effect a positive outcome.

Cost is a consideration just as important as proper delivery mechanism. Powdered herbs, including concentrates of appropriate herbs, generally prove to be the best bargain. The cost to your patient for a therapeutic dosage for regular tablets is between $1.00 and $2.20 per day. Daily cost for teas is usually between $2.50 to $3.50.

Commercial tinctures use six pounds of herbal matter per gallon of extracting liquid. This translates to 42 grams of herbs per two ounce tincture. Standard retail cost for a two ounce tincture is from $13.00 to $44.00. This works out to a lowest cost of 31 cents per gram. A typical bottle of pills, however, will contain 90 tablets weighing .75 grams each for a total weight of 67.5 grams. At $16.00 retail per bottle the cost is 23.7 cents per gram. It should be remembered that a two ounce tincture is an extraction from 42 grams of herbs before ingestion, whereas tableting provides the herbs directly for ingestion.

There is much more to the prescribing of herbs than just the selection of the proper formula. The form in which the herbs are ingested is an extremely important consideration in the treatment of your patients. This makes the manufacturing process just as important.

Although in some cases American practitioners can obtain products manufactured in China, these are generally not recommended because of erratic labeling, poor quality, and the possibility that pharmaceutical drugs may be in these products. Well known products such as Yin Chao frequently contain caffeine and antihistamines, while products for arthritis have been discovered to have various prescription and non-prescription drugs. Stress aids can contain Cinnabar, a toxic mercury compound.

The highest quality herbs in China are exported, which is why many practitioners from China are impressed by the herbs obtained in America. As a rule, products manufactured in the U.S. offer higher quality controls than those manufactured in China. Since higher quality herbs are used the dosage is lower. Products manufactured in the U.S. contain pure herbs without fillers, artificial dyes, or other unnatural ingredients.

We have offered some arguments for and against the various forms of prescribing herbs. However, physician and commentator Sima Qian of the Han dynasty and author of the *Annals of History*, should have the last word: "What people suffer from is a multitude of illnesses; what physicians suffer from is a paucity of approaches."*

Forgotten Traditions of Ancient Chinese Medicine by Paul Unschuld, Paradigm Publications. Brookline, MA. 1990

Chinese Dietary Therapy

Chinese food therapy is based on the principle of eating a variety of foods according to one's own constitution. There is no single best diet for everyone. Our rates of metabolism are different, the climates that we live in vary, and our amounts of exercise differ. Furthermore, we all have different health patterns — some individuals are never ill, while others are frequently so, and the body sites that are affected by the same pathogen may be different in different persons.

Chinese dietary principles

In this society of abundance, there is no reason to eat only fruits, or only vegetables, or to eat the same foods day-in and day-out. Ideally, one should primarily consume cooked vegetables and cooked grains. These are an excellent source of fiber and nutrition. In terms of grains, rice, the staple of Asian diet, is an excellent food as it is easy to digest and is neither too hot nor too cold energetically. Other suitable staple foods include potatoes, sweet potatoes, millet, and the like.

From a Chinese energetic perspective, there is nothing wrong with a small amount of meat once a day. Even Tibetan Buddhist monks who believe in the sanctity of all living creatures eat meat occasionally in order to sustain warmth against the harsh Himalayan winters. In this fast-paced world, most people have busy lives with demanding schedules, and need the energy and nutrition that meats provide. Although it is possible to obtain adequate nutrition as a vegetarian, most individuals in our society are not proper vegetarians. Many Americans in their attempt to reduce or eliminate meat from their diet actually end up eating an excess of dairy products in the form yogurt, cheese, and milk. According to Chinese dietary principles, only children should consume milk. One of the common energetic imbalances is a preponderance of Dampness. Dairy products, in addition to being highly allergenic substances, are not suitable for individuals with this type of imbalance and should be avoided. In particular, cheese is too warm in property and also produces Dampness. Thus, for individuals with a Dampness pattern, they may be healthier by eating meat or by learning how to correctly obtain protein from vegetable sources rather than relying so heavily on dairy products.

Another Chinese dietary principle is that all food should be eaten while it is warm or hot. In order to utilize food for energy, the body must first bring it to body temperature. Thus, if food is consumed while hot, the body can immediately transform it into energy. This is why drinks with ice, or those consumed upon removal from the refrigerator, should be avoided. Preferably, all beverages should be consumed hot, even water, although this is not always practical. When eating out, request beverages without ice, and at home simply do not put ice in drinks, or allow refrigerated ones to come to room temperature before drinking. Since liquids facilitate the transformation of food into energy, hot water or herbal tea should be taken with meals. Cooking of food actually helps in its being digested since the heating process breaks down the cellulose cell walls of vegetables where most of the vitamins and nutrients are located. By eating mainly warm or hot food, one will feel more energetic, and have fewer digestive complaints.

Another aspect of Chinese diet, which is common to many spiritual traditions, is chewing food carefully. Most individuals chew inattentively and then gulp their food down with liquids. By taking time to chew (usually seven or more times for each bite), digestion is enhanced, as is the enjoyment of the food. Mealtimes should be relaxed and without pressure to finish. The Chinese also advocate eating in season. For healthy persons, this means that when the climate is cold, hot food should be taken, and when the weather is warm, the food temperature may be cooler. Individuals who are not in good health should eat hot food only. Fruits should be eaten in their whole forms, and should not be consumed as juices since the latter are too concentrated.

Ancient wisdom

Li Dongguan, a famous physician of the Jin dynasty, stated that the primordial Qi of the Spleen and Stomach is the foundation of life. Pathogenic injury of the Spleen and Stomach can cause various diseases. Li advocated restraint in food and drink, eating cereals more than meat, being content with life without fame and wealth, and shunning worry and desire. To cultivate the primordial Qi, one should keep warm and avoid wind, cold, and overexertion. Chen Zhongling of the Qing dynasty indicated in his *Four Essentials of Health Preservation* to eat and drink in moderation, avoid invasion of Wind and Cold, "spare the mind," and to shun anger. According to Chinese medicine, if the mind is not calm, problems with the circulation of Qi and Blood will arise. Perhaps one would do well to bear in mind the Chinese adage, "Laughter makes one ten years younger, distress causes one's hair to become grey, and anger hastens one's death." A renowned Chinese poet once wrote, ". . . with the spirit improved and the mind in a pleasant frame, disease can be cured."

Tea

Americans drink enormous amounts of coffee. However, not only is caffeine a stimulant with immediate effects, it also overstimulates the adrenal gland, which leads to a delayed feeling of fatigue. Furthermore, the acids in coffee can cause digestive problems. In Chinese medicine, coffee is known to be sweet and warm in properties, which is why many coffee drinkers have a preponderance of Dampness in their system. On the other hand, tea is slightly bitter and cool in properties, thus making it an important component of Chinese (and Asian) diet. There are several kinds of tea, the more common of which are green, black, and scented. Green tea is cool in property; it is capable of reducing fever and is taken in the summer. Black tea warms the Spleen and Stomach and is particularly suitable to drink in winter. Scented teas, such as jasmine, may be taken during all seasons. The Tang dynasty poet, Lu Tong, once wrote, "Seven bowls of tea bring seven advantages: One, it promotes the production of body fluids and quenches thirst; two, it refreshes the mind; three, it helps digestion; four, it induces sweating to relieve the common cold; five, it helps fat people reduce weight; six, it activates thinking and strengthens memory; and seven, it ensures longevity."

Dietary guidelines

Dietary changes should be introduced slowly, so as not to cause imbalance or exacerbate existing conditions. Too-rapid dietary changes may even bring on new illnesses. To go too quickly from a high protein and/or junk food diet to one that consists mainly of vegetables and grains is unwise. It is also important to avoid overeating; a better method is to eat smaller quantities more frequently, and to stop eating before one is full. Breakfast and lunch should be the main meals, and dinner just a light repast.

The following are guidelines according to Chinese dietary principles that may be helpful in improving one's diet and health.

Foods and beverages that should be avoided:

Alcohol (except individuals with Cold patterns)
Raw foods (except during summer months or in warm climates)
Junk food
Greasy and fried foods
Sweets and diet foods
Ice cold foods and beverages
Fruit juices

Common Food Allergens:

Corn
Wheat
Soy
Chocolate
Tomatoes and tomato products
Citrus fruits and juices
Dairy products

Recommended foods and beverages:

Lean meat or fish — 2 oz per day
Vegetables — fresh, lightly cooked or stir-fried, with skins retained (skinless for irritable bowel sufferers)
Eggs — in moderation
Fruits — whole (candidiasis sufferers may need to avoid)
Grains — should be mainstay of diet
Rice
Whole grains (if not allergenic)
    Millet
    Wheat (if not allergenic)
    Buckwheat
    Corn (if not allergenic)
    Oats
Beans and peas
Stews, casseroles, soups

Foods that may need evaluation:

Soy products
Yeast-containing foods
Fermented foods, vinegar
Nuts
Cereals (may exacerbate digestive conditions)
Spicy foods
Citrus fruits
Tomato products
Shellfish

Chinese vs. Western Herbology

Compared with Western herbal medicine, Chinese herbal medicine is more complex, more complete, and used by a greater number of people. In Western herbal medicine there is no systematic practice, although accumulated experience has discovered individual herbs, such as echinacea, goldenseal, and crampbark, that have excellent properties. Since there is little in the way of formal training, Western herbalists gravitate towards individual teachers or schools. With few exceptions, Western herbalists are influenced primarily by the "folk" tradition rather then medical practice, and relatively little is known about the effects of herbal combinations. Most Western herbalists see far fewer patients than do trained Chinese herbalists.

Chinese herbology, on the other hand, has developed from a three-thousand year-old practice. Textbooks such as the *Sha Hun Lun*, written 1800 years ago, are still used today. The herbal formulas contained in this book are frequently prescribed every day in China, Japan, and the United States. Each major city in China has a traditional hospital, where cases of such serious conditions as heart disease, viral infection, and stroke are treated exclusively with acupuncture and herbal medicine. Furthermore, research efforts have concentrated on integrating Chinese and Western medicine, such as with cancer patients who receive chemotherapy and radiotherapy along with herbs that offset the side effects of these treatments. Associated with each hospital is an academy where students are fully trained and eventually specialize in particular areas of herbal medicine.

A typical successful Chinese herbalist in America is someone who has had ten to sixty years' experience. A practitioner like Dr. Fung in Oakland, California, regularly sees fifty to a hundred patients per day, has had sixty years' experience, has run hospital wards where herbal medicine was practiced, and regularly prescribes at least five hundred herbs.

Important Herbal Tips

1. Herbs should not be used during pregnancy except under the direction of an experienced herbalist.

2. Tonic herbs or formulas are inappropriate during the initial stages of a cold or flu. In addition to making the body stronger, tonics may also make the cold or flu stronger. Instead, use specific cold and flu herbal formulas and resume tonic formulas once the illness has run its course.

3. Herbs are inappripriate during menstruation except for acute symptoms. For example, cold and flu treatments can be administered. Specific formulas for menstrual cramps or nausea can also be administered.

4. If you get no response within a few days in an acute condition, or within a month for a chronic condition, you should probably use another formula or consult a more experienced herbalist. Be sure the patient has been taking an adequate dose, usually at least nine tablets a day for a chronic condition, or more for an acute condition. It is not unusual for herbs to be taken every few hours for acute conditions, or up to 20 tablets a day for chronic conditions. If the herbs are working, the patient should at least feel better after this period, even if the condition is not gone.

5. Approximately one percent of American patients have allergies to one or more Chinese herbs. Patients with excess Dampness need to have the Dampness reduced before they can tolerate some herbs, particularly tonics. Ten percent of seriously ill patients cannot tolerate Chinese herbs. In many cases these patients severely underdose to the point where the herbs cannot give any benefit.

6. Patients who have food allergies or digestive problems, or who seem unusually sensitive, need to be started at a lower dose of herbs and gradually built up to an normal dose. In such cases, herbs can also be taken with meals or combined with a digestive formula such as Quiet Digestion.

7. Pharmaceutical drugs, recreational drugs, and vitamin supplements tend to be warming and contribute to Yin deficiency. Excessive coffee, dairy, alcohol, sweets, greasy and fried foods, and meats — all typical of a Western diet — tend to cause Damp Heat. Formulas such as

Phellostatin are excellent to use on a long-term basis when patients suffer from the combined effects of Dampness and Heat.

8. If you are sure your diagnosis is accurate and you are not getting adequate results with a formula, keep in mind that even slight variations in formulas may produce better results in some patients. In chronic conditions there is often Blood stagnation; therefore a formula such as Flavonex, which activates Blood, can be used as an adjunct for chronic conditions. Chronic conditions also usually involve deficiency and excess conditions, and both Yin and Yang deficiency; therefore use a balanced formula. If patients have mixed Hot and Cold signs it is also important to use a balanced formula. Astra Essence and Astra Isatis, both balanced formulas, are frequently used for this reason.

9. Patients who have not taken herbs before usually need a smaller dose than those who have taken herbs over a long period. Those who have taken herbs regularly probably need to exceed the recommended dose. Recommended dosages are for adults in the 100-200 lb. range. Some practitioners recommend lower dosages for children; others recommend the adult dosage for children over the age of five. Children generally have strong Yang energy and have no problems absorbing and utilizing adult doses of herbs.

10. Some patients, particularly those with autoimmune diseases, will turn rapidly from a Cold pattern to a Heat pattern or vice versa. Therefor they must be continually monitored and treated accordingly. Other patients may present with one pattern in the morning and a different pattern in another part of the day. With these patients it is not unusual to give them a warming formula in one part of the day and cooling formula to take in another part of the day.

To the patient

This book is not designed for self treatment without the guidance of a practitioner. Many of these formulas are not available over-the-counter or through mail order. They must be obtained as prepared formulas through a practitioner, or in decoction form from an herbalist in Chinatown. Chinese herbs work in a hit-or-miss fashion when they are used according to Western medicine without regard to Traditional Chinese Medicine, so you will need a trained practitioner to make the proper diagnosis in terms of Chinese medicine. Most licensed or registered acupuncturists are qualified to diagnose according to Chinese medicine, and can supply these formulas. In some cases patients may harm themselves by using Chinese herbs inappropriately. Particularly when one is chronically ill, it is extremely difficult to see the forest for the trees. A practitioner can perform the valuable service of giving perspective on one's health, and offering valuable suggestions such as lifestyle and dietary modifications, which are necessary to get the most from herbal therapy. For the best care of the patient, the suggestions indicated in this book are meant to be combined with Western medicine, and this book should never be used as the sole basis for recommending treatment.

Addictions

Western Medicine

Alcohol, drug, and nicotine addictions are rampant throughout the Western world. Twelve Step and other support therapies seem to be very effective. Acupuncture is also gaining recognition as a successful component in the treatment of addictions. Coffee is an addictive substance that can harm the digestive system and can contribute to high blood pressure.

TCM

With alcoholism there is stagnant Liver Qi, usually with Heat. Nicotine addiction introduces a tremendous amount of Heat to the Lung, and also weakens the Lung. Most drugs deplete the Yin and create Shen disturbance. Marijuana also destroys the Spleen. Coffee causes Damp Heat in the Spleen, Stomach, and Intestines.

Chinese Herbal Therapy

Chinese therapy is meant as an adjunct to acupuncture and Twelve Step programs. Good results can be expected, keeping in mind that herbs help the body cope with withdrawal. Ease Plus, based on the traditional formula Bupleurum and Dragonbone, has been used for more than ten years in the U.S. for addiction. It contains herbs which sedate the Shen, improve the digestive system, and remove Heat. Ginseng in this formula tonifies the Spleen.

In many cases I have found the Schizandra Dreams formula to be more effective, because nearly all the herbs in the formula are sedating. The dose is three to five tablets whenever the patient feels anxious. I began to recommend this formula after some patients either did not take enough Ease Plus to give noticeable effects, or who took too much and became too sedated.

Nicotine

For long-term smokers, Clear Air is an excellent formula to relieve the chest. Initial therapy may begin with either Ease Plus or Schizandra Dreams, or both if the patient has insomnia. After two to four weeks, Clear Air may be used to ventilate the Lung. The usual course of treatment is one to three months. If there is dryness of the Lung, an excellent formula is Wise Judge, based on Glenia Ophiopogonis Drink (Sha Shen Mai Dong Yin) and Generate the Pulse Powder (Sheng Mai San). This formula is also recommended after a fever or for upper respiratory problems.

Schizandra Dreams
Kava Kava Formula

Ingredients

English	Latin/*pinyin*
Kava Kava	Piper methysticum
Schizandra	Wu Wei Zi
Oystershell	Mu Li
Dragonbone	Long Gu
Amber	Hu Po

(see also: Ease Plus, Clear Air, Wise Judge, Ecliptex, Calm Spirit, Six Gentlemen, Source Qi)

Alcohol

For alcoholism, include Ecliptex with Ease Plus or Schizandra Dreams. Ecliptex helps repair damage done to the Liver. It should probably be taken for a year or more by the alcoholic.

Cocaine/Marijuana

For cocaine addiction, Calm Spirit is an excellent formula since cocaine seems to create a lot of Heat in the Heart. Marijuana addicts may need treatment similar to that for nicotine addicts (see above) or Six Gentlemen to tonify the Spleen and clear up Spleen Dampness. In either case Ease Plus or Schizandra Dreams should be used during the initial withdrawal phase. Those addicted to drugs may also benefit by taking Ecliptex to repair the Liver.

Caffeine

Those wishing to cut down on coffee or other caffeinated beverages can try taking two to three tablets of Adrenosen for an energy burst. Adrenosen does not have the rebound depression associated with coffee drinking.

Case Studies
Case 1
A man in his mid forties, addicted to cocaine, was given Ease Plus by his practitioner. The patient reported that if he took three tablets of Ease Plus TID, nothing happened. When his practitioner told him to increase to four or five tablets TID, he reported he was "too zonked out."

I suggested taking Schizandra Dreams, three tablets TID. He reported that this formula effectively cut the "jitters" or nervousness associated with cocaine withdrawal. This patient was also receiving acupuncture, although only once a week.

Case 2
A female patient in her late thirties, addicted to coffee, was having frequent gas, bloating, and diarrhea, and fatigue after eating lunch. The tongue was usually pale, although it sometimes showed Heat; her pulse was slow and weak. She was reluctant to give up coffee, and after only moderate success with Quiet Digestion, I persuaded her to cut down to one cup of coffee a day, substituting black tea and two tablets of Adrenosen daily. I also gave her the Source Qi formula. After two days, all her symptoms were alleviated.

Allergic Rhinitis (Hayfever)

Western Medicine

Most people with hayfever have taken over-the-counter or prescription medications for the condition. Some of these contain ephedrine or pseudoephedrine which were initially synthesized from the chinese herb Ma Huang. Allergy shots are also common.

TCM

Wind Invading Nose, which can be caused by Kidney or Spleen deficiency; Excess Phlegm.

Chinese Herbal Therapy

Treatment can be effective, but usually involves multiple therapies. For acute symptoms I have clients take two tablets of Xanthium Relieve Surface and one tablet of Astra C. Astra C is used to increase the Wei Qi (defensive energy). Usually results are seen within ten minutes. If there are no results within a half-hour, repeat the dose. This combination can be taken throughout the day. It does not cause drowsiness or irritation.

If the phlegm is colored, Nasal Tabs may provide faster relief. However this formula contains Ma Huang and may be too stimulating to some patients, in which case the Xanthium Relieve Surface may still be used.

For individuals with simultaneous digestive problems, Quiet Digestion is an excellent adjunct to Xanthium Relieve Surface.

The patient's Wei Qi, or defensive energy, must be built up to protect against Wind attack. Astra C, based on the Jade Screen formula, with vitamin C and zinc, is an excellent choice; vitamin C has been said to reduce allergy symptoms. Best results may be obtained by taking Astra C before the allergy season begins. Royal Jelly also maybe used in order to build up defensive energy.

Therefore, typical therapy may involve using Astra C or Royal Jelly every day a few months before the allergy season begins, then taking Xanthium Relieve Surface with Astra C until it relieves symptoms.

Another excellent formula is Six Gentlemen, to be used preventively with Astra C, particularly if there is low energy, loose stools, and watery diarrhea.

Notes

It is essential that dairy products be eliminated. Patients should adopt a TCM diet.

Case Study

A man in his thirties had allergic rhinitis ever since he could remember. He had a slow pulse and a pale tongue. He'd had allergy shots as a child, and had tried various herbal or homeopathic remedies from Chinese pharmacies and health food stores. These had either worked and then stopped working several weeks later, or had provided no substantial relief. He was given Xanthium Relieve Surface. A three tablet dose produced no results, but five tablets at once alleviated the hayfever for a few hours, after which it flared back up. Once a week he still needed to use an over-the-counter remedy to control the symptoms.

When two tablets of Quiet Digestion were added to each dose of Xanthium Relieve Surface, his eyes no longer watered, he was able to reduce the dosage of Xanthium Relieve Surface, and he had to use the over-the-counter remedy even less.

Xanthium Relieve Surface

Ingredients

English	pinyin
Xanthium	Cang Er Zi
Chrysanthemum	Ju Hua
Astragalus	Huang Qi
Ligusticum	Chuan Xiong
Schizonepeta	Jing Jie
Phellodendron	Huang Bai
Siler	Fang Feng
Angelica	Bai Zhi
Rehmannia	Shu Di Huang
Mume	Wu Mei
Platycodon	Jie Geng
Asarum	Xi Xin
Anemarrhena	Zhi Mu
Licorice	Gan Cao

(see also: Quiet Digestion, Nasal Tabs, Astra C, Flavonex)

A few weeks later, when the symptoms abated due to less pollen in the air, I used Six Gentlemen formula as a tonic, and his general energy level improved. After taking various tonic formulas including Shen-Gem for a period when he was under stress, Astra C during the cold and flu season (he was subject to repeated colds and flu) and Astra Essence for frequent urination, he reported significantly less hayfever and less dependence on over-the-counter medications the following spring.

Amenorrhea

Western Medicine

Primary amenorrhea refers to women over the age of sixteen who have never menstruated. Secondary amenorrhea refers to women who have not menstruated for three months. Because either form of amenorrhea can be secondary to other conditions, a complete medical workup and gynecological exam is indicated.

TCM

Treatment is usually not suitable for primary amenorrhea, but can be effective for the secondary type. Secondary amenorrhea is usually due to either Spleen and Kidney deficiency, Qi and Blood deficiency, or Blood stasis with Cold.

Chinese Herbal Therapy

For Spleen and Kidney deficiency Astra Essence can be used. For additional Spleen tonification it can be combined with Six Gentlemen. If there is a gradual loss of menstruation accompanied by dizziness, short breath, pale complexion, and pale tongue, Eight Treasures is an excellent formula. For Blood stasis with Cold and Qi stagnation, use Crampbark Plus.

Case Studies

Case 1

A woman in her early twenties hadn't menstruated for one year. It is interesting to note that in many respects she looked like and acted like a teenager. She was a dancer, and possibly anorectic or bulimic, although this was just a hunch.

I told her to take a combination of Astra Essence and Eight Treasures, two tablets of each TID. After three months she began spotting. She also had more color in the face and reported more energy.

Case 2

A nineteen year-old woman with anorectic appearance, also anemic, said that it had been six months since she had her period. The tongue was pale and the pulse was slow. Initially I put her on Eight Treasures, 3 tablets TID. After approximately four weeks there was essentially no change, so I told her to combine 2 tablets Eight Treasures and 2 tablets Astra Essence TID.

After another two months she had scant menstruation. I advised her to continue the second protocol for at least six months, if not longer.

Analysis: My first attempt at building up the Blood was probably not enough, as this patient seemed to be unusually thin and lacking muscle tone. Astra Essence helps build up Kidney Jing, Yin and Yang whereas the Eight Treasures primarily builds up Qi and Blood.

Astra Essence
Restorative Herbal Formula

Ingredients

English	pinyin
Astragalus root/seed	Huang Qi/Sha Yuan Ji Zi
Ligustrum	Nu Zhen Zi
Ho-shou-wu	He Shou Wu
Lycium fruit	Gou Qi Zi
Rehmannia	Shu Di Huang
Eucommia	Du Zhong
Cuscuta	Tu Si Zi
Ginseng	Ren Shen
Tang-kuei	Dang Gui
Cornus	Shan Zhu Yu

(see also: Six Gentlemen, Eight Treasures, Woman's Precious, Crampbark Plus)

Anemia and Leukopenia

Western Medicine

Anemia is an abnormally low red blood cell count; Leukopenia is an abnormally low white blood cell count.

TCM

Anemia is usually treated with Blood tonic herbs. Treatment of leukopenia usually involves Spleen tonification.

Chinese Herbal Therapy

I helped develop Marrow Plus, based on research work done at Quan Yin Clinic in San Francisco, to treat drug-induced anemia due to agents such as AZT, chemotherapy and radiation therapy, or to regenerate blood following blood transfusions. This formula may also be used for neuropathy as well as with other anemias.

Marrow Plus contains herbs that tonify and invigorate Blood and strengthen the Spleen and Kidney. The main ingredient is Milletia (Ji Xue Tang), which is the chief herb in Chinese research formulas for treating anemia. This formula can be combined with Back-

Marrow Plus
Milletia Herbal Formula

Ingredients

English	pinyin
Milletia	Ji Xue Teng
Ho-shou-wu	He Shou Wu
Salvia	Dan Shen
Codonopsis	Dang Shen
Astragalus	Huang Qi
Ligusticum	Chuan Xiong
Raw Rehmannia	Sheng Di Huang
Cooked Rehmannia	Shu Di Huang
Lycium	Gou Ji Zi
Tang-kuei	Dang Gui
Lotus Seed	Lian Zi
Citrus	Chen Pi
Red Date Extract	Da Zao
Oryza	Gu Ya
Gelatinum	E Jiao

(see also: Astra 8, Backbone, Eight Treasures)

bone, which tonifies Kidney Yang, in order to get a stronger and more immediate effect, however, the patients must have a Cold condition since Backbone is a warming formula.

Marrow Plus can also be used for leukopenia, but good results have also been achieved with Astra 8, which is more of a Spleen tonic. Marrow Plus will also potentiate iron supplementation. To tonify both Qi and Blood, use Eight Treasures.

Case Study

A woman in her forties with a long history of leukopenia was administered Astra 8, and eight weeks later she reported that her white blood count was approaching the normal range.

Arthritis

Western Medicine
Arthritis is the inflammation of a joint, usually accompanied by pain, swelling, and structural changes. Arthritis is linked to infection, rheumatic fever, ulcerative colitis, trauma, neurogenic disturbance, degenerative joint disease such as osteoarthritis, metabolic disturbance such as gout, psoriasis, Raynaud's syndrome, bursitis, etc.

Complications of Western Medications
This is a difficult condition to treat, and cases are usually complicated by treatment with Western drugs, such as non-steroidal anti-inflammatory-drugs (NSAID), or steroids. Aspirin and other NSAID may weaken the digestive system so that Quiet Digestion or Stomach Tabs are necessary. Steroids damage the Kidney and therefore a formula such as Astra Essence may be used to give the Kidney more energy.

TCM
Arthritis is usually caused by Wind, Cold, and Dampness, accompanied by obstruction of Qi and Blood. However, there are cases of acute attacks following infections that are caused by Yin deficiency with internal Heat. Heat is a prominent characteristic in all acute attacks of Rheumatoid arthritis. Sea Cucumber is also recommended by traditional herbalists for joint pain. It is available as a food or in tablets.

Chinese Herbal Therapy
Mobility 2 is based on the ancient formula Shu Jing Huo Xue Tang (Clematis and Stephania Formula). This formula dispels Wind, Dampness, and Cold. It also vitalizes the Blood and contains tonic herbs and therefore can be taken long-term for those who have weakened constitutions. It also has anti-inflammatory properties.

AC-Q is used to treat arthritis, and contains a number of aromatic herbs which are especially good for eliminating Dampness. Therefore practitioners in damp or humid environments report this formula is more effective. It may also be used when there are pus-filled swellings, or with pain characterized as aching, as it contains Qi moving herbs.

In severe cases AC-Q and Mobility 2 may be combined, using two tablets of each formula TID or QID.

Dr. Fung's Mobility 3 is used for Wind and for Damp Cold pain. It is based on his 60 years' experience with Chinese herbs.

Mobility 2
Clematis and Stephania Combination
(Shu Jing Huo Xue Tang)

Ingredients

English	pinyin
Red Peony	Chi Shao
Tang-kuei	Dang Gui
Cnidium	Chuan Xiong
Rehmannia	Shu Di Huang
Persica	Tao Ren
Atractylodes	Bai Zhu
Poria	Fu Ling
Siler	Fang Feng
Citrus	Chen Pi
Stephania	Fang Ji
Gentiana	Long Dan Cao
Achyranthes	Niu Xi
Chiang-huo	Qiang Huo
Clematis	Wei Ling Xian
Ginger	Gan Jiang
Angelica	Bai Zhi
Licorice	Gan Cao

(see also: Meridian Circulation, Mobility 3, AC-Q, Flavonex, Backbone, Coptis Purge Fire, Resinall K)

Flavonex is a modern formula containing anti-inflammatory flavonoids. It contains herbs which nourish circulation, and therefore this is often an excellent adjunct formula. Flavonex may also be used if there is Heat, as it is not overly warming. Coptis Purge Fire can be used if there is internal Heat, for example to reduce the burning in the initial stages of gout. It is recommended to be taken with Nine Flavor Tea, which will promote diuresis and take Heat out of the Blood. Suggested dosage is two tablets of each formula every two to three hours combined with Western medicine. Coptis Purge Fire tablets can also be crushed and applied topically as a wash mixed with water. The above formulas may need to be directed by using Head-Q for upper body gout, whereas Mobility 2 could be used for lower body gout. While the short-term strategy involves clearing Heat, the long-term management of gout involves adopting a low purine diet, abstaining from alcohol, and using constitutional formulas such as Nine Flavor Tea with Yin deficiency, Six Gentlemen for Qi deficiency, or Rehmannia 8 for Yang deficiency.

Backbone is for a weak back and weak bones caused by Kidney Yang deficiency. Resinall K may be used for arthritis caused by trauma. It is a liquid extract and should be held under the tongue.

Notes

It is important for those who have arthritis to maintain a diet eliminating raw foods, fried foods, and iced or cold foods and drinks. Alcohol in moderation may be beneficial because it is warming.

Case Studies

Case 1

A thirty year-old female patient diagnosed with rheumatoid arthritis, with a red tongue, fast pulse and tremendous pain in all her joints, taking cortisone and several other medications, got 50-60% pain reduction a few days after taking Clear Heat. The pain reduction lasted for a month, and then pain began to return. My suggestion was to take AC-Q, as I have gotten very good results with joint pain, particularly in the lower body. I also recommended Nine Flavor Tea, since it was my belief that the medications were causing Yin deficiency, which was the cause of the Heat signs. Also the disease itself was causing Heat signs, as it is an inflammatory condition. Suggested dosage was two tablets of each formula QID.

Case 2

A woman in her seventies with chronic osteoarthritis had definite signs of osteoporosis, edema, obesity, digestive troubles, and pale tongue. Her rapid pulse may have been caused by the several prescription medications she was taking. She reported that her medications just weren't working as they had in the past, and she was trying to avoid being put on a higher dosage of corticosteroids.

Since she was in such a high level of pain, I suggested combining Mobility 2, two tablets TID, with two tablets of AC-Q TID. I said if she did not get relief, she could increase the dosage of Mobility 2. I also told her to take Quiet Digestion any time she ate a big meal or had other digestive discomfort (she had reported that big meals "got stuck in her intestines").

The patient reported significant pain relief within a week of taking the herbs. She wanted to start taking formulas for weight loss. However, I thought it was best to keep her on the combination of AC-Q and Mobility 2 for the next several weeks.

Analysis: There have been many patients who have had chronic arthritis who haven't responded to Mobility 2 alone, which is why I almost always use a combination of formulas. It is very common for arthritis patients, even those who get good results, to lose interest in the Chinese herbs after several weeks or months, as they are anxious to try other therapies.

Case 3

A woman in her early sixties complained of hand and finger arthritis that was so severe that the pain and swelling was only relieved by cortisone injections. She had suffered this way for several years. She was put on Mobility 2 by her practitioner and after two weeks there was considerably less pain and greater movement. After six months on Mobility 2 she was pleased with the results. Mobility 2 is a good general formula as it addresses the major components of chronic arthritis including Blood stasis, Dampness, and Wind.

Asthma, Bronchitis
Bronchial Asthma,
Chronic Bronchitis, Emphysema

Western Medicine

Asthma involves recurrent attacks of shortness of breath, wheezing, and expectoration of phlegm. Medical treatment often involves the use of bronchial dilators. Note that bronchial dilators can mask the true nature of the disorder. Steroid medications may also be prescribed, and these may lead to Kidney deficiency.

TCM

It is necessary to differentiate between Hot and Cold patterns. Treatment must also include ventilating the Lung, eliminating Phlegm, correcting underlying deficiency.

Chinese Herbal Therapy

Treatment usually involves an acute formula and a constitutional formula. The acute formulas include Minor Blue Dragon, a traditional formula that addresses Phlegm that is watery or white, or tearing; and Clear Air, which is a modification of Ding Chuan Tang, and is for colored, yellow, or green phlegm. If there is a weakness of the Lung and Spleen, characterized by weak cough, shortness of breath, tendency to catch cold, loose stools, whitish tongue coat, the Astra 8 formula has been very successful. If there are chronic or recurrent asthma attacks over a long period of time, and constant persistent asthma, the Ginseng and Gecko formula is an excellent choice; it addresses Lung deficiency with Heat and helps the Kidney grasp the Qi of the Lung. Isatis Gold may be used in the initial stage of bronchitis. If the patient has taken steroids, evaluate Astra Essence or Ginseng and Gecko Formula.

Notes

TCM diet; fresh ginger tea is good for Cold signs; watermelon is said to be good with Heat signs; walnuts and figs are also said to benefit asthma. Eliminate dairy products completely.

Case Studies

Case 1

A woman in her sixties had severe asthma and fatigue, which disabled her to the point that she couldn't leave the house, even to do her grocery shopping. A colleague put her on Ginseng and Gecko and after one month her breathing and fatigue greatly improved, so that she was able to do grocery shopping for the first time in several years.

Ginseng and Gecko

Ingredients

English	*pinyin*
Apricot Seed	Ku Xing Ren
Baked Licorice	Zhi Gan Cao
White Ginseng	Ren Shen
Poria	Fu Ling
Morus Bark	Sang Bai Pi
Fritillaria Bulb	Chuan Bei Mu
Anemarrhena	Zhi Mu
Gecko	Ge Jie

(see also: Minor Blue Dragon, Clear Air, Astra 8, Isatis Gold, Wise Judge, Lucid Channel)

Case 2

A woman in her mid-thirties developed severe asthma after a bad case of bronchitis. She was having a severe asthma attack every day. The patient usually had copious clear nasal discharge. She was put on bulk herbs to control the symptoms. The patient initially came in because she was trying to get pregnant and hadn't been able to conceive. Her condition improved dramatically when the practitioner added Ginseng and Gecko formula in pill form, along with bulk herbs. One year later the patient got pregnant, and now has only mild wheezing.

Analysis: Ginseng and Gecko is a formula for chronic asthma, and is to be used as a constitutional formula. It is usually used for several months to address weak Lung, Dampness, and Spleen and Kidney deficiency. Therefore it is best to use bulk herbs or a prepared formula such as Minor Blue Dragon for Cold signs, and Clear Air for Heat signs. Isatis Gold has given good results with acute bronchitis. Infertility may also be due to Kidney Yang deficiency, and therefore the Ginseng and Gecko formula also helped treat her infertility.

Case 3

A thirty year-old female runner came in complaining of asthmatic breathing, digestive disorders, and fatigue. For five years she had run five to ten miles a day, and worked out with weights several times per week. She was mostly vegetarian, but sometimes ate chicken. I first asked her if she ate any dairy products and she said that she had cereal every morning. I suggested that she eliminate cereal as a breakfast, and she told me that she would just as soon die as not eat cereal. This troubled me, because people are often addicted to their worst-offending foods. Cereal is difficult for many people to digest, and I have read reports that those with chronic digestive disorders frequently are cereal eaters. Milk of course is an offending agent, but the corn and wheat present in many cereals can also be allergens. I strongly suggested that this client cut out cereal for just two weeks to see if there was an improvement in her bronchial and digestive systems. She still did not seem willing, so I suggested switching to soy milk, or better, rice milk.

She had pale skin and a pale tongue, and a rapid to normal pulse. Seemingly healthy competitive athletes often deplete their Essence through their excessive exercise. She reported that she often missed her menstrual period, which is further evidence of this.

I put her on Ginseng and Gecko formula, Minor Blue Dragon, and Quiet Digestion before eating dairy products or when her stomach was "acting up." I had initially put her on two tablets of Ginseng and Gecko, and two tablets of Minor Blue Dragon TID. My strategy was to withdraw the Minor Blue Dragon after one or two bottles and follow up with Kidney or Blood tonics.

After two weeks she reported a slight improvement in her digestive system, and "perhaps slight improvement in the fatigue, not really sure, no change in the asthma." She had also started taking Echinacea, which was recommended at a health food store. I told her to stop taking the Echinacea and save it for when she got a cold or flu, since it is not appropriate for long-term use (more than ten days) according to Western herbalists. There had been no change in her tongue and pulse.

She kept taking the Chinese herbs but, although her fatigue began to improve, the asthma showed only a slight change; Quiet Digestion seemed to help the acute digestive disorders. Six weeks after beginning the herbs, the patient decided to leave the area, and I referred her to a practitioner where she was living.

Analysis: The patient was put on Ginseng and Gecko, since her copious phlegm was often colored, and because she had taken Western medication for several months for pneumonia. Colored phlegm indicates Heat and Western drugs are almost always Heat-producing. She also had many Cold symptoms, including always feeling cold, and sometimes her phlegm was clear, so I felt Minor Blue Dragon might be good to drive out the exterior Cold. Clear Air is usually the companion to Ginseng and Gecko. If I had continued treatment I most likely would have had her continue taking the Ginseng and Gecko, and would have substituted Astra Essence for the Minor Blue Dragon, which was not symptomatically improving the lungs as I had thought. I also might have tried Clear Air.

Traditionally, Ginseng and Gecko is given for several months before the condition improves, although I have seen severe asthmatic patients literally turn their life around after several weeks on this formula. Most of my lifestyle advice had been discarded: eating more meat, quitting dairy products, especially milk, eliminating salads in favor of warm foods, and considering running every other day until her health improved. I attribute the lack of more dramatic progress to this. Even though only slight gains were made, the client was willing to continue taking the herbs, although I had a feeling she never took as many as I suggested.

Case 4

A young acupuncture student came to me with severe asthma; she took inhalant medications, (twice a day, down from one every few hours) which she was hoping to stop. She had been able to discontinue her steroid medication through weekly acupuncture treatments, but not the inhaler. I asked what kind of phlegm she had (which is an important indicator as to whether there are Hot or Cold signs) and she said she had almost no phlegm, which I then guessed was a side effect of the inhaler. This patient said on the rare occasion she did have phlegm it was colored, suggesting Heat. The patient also was very tired, pale, and slightly overweight, indicating Dampness. The patient had used Lung Yin tonics but they were not helping. I suggested taking the Ginseng and Gecko formula since it would help build up the Kidney in addition to clearing Heat from the Lung, with the Clear Air formula, which I hoped would noticeably improve her breathing. I told her to use the Ginseng and Gecko formula cautiously, since it is traditionally indicated for a productive cough. Thus she took two tablets of Clear Air and one tablet of Ginseng and Gecko TID. I told her to increase the Ginseng and Gecko by one tablet the second week if she was doing well. I suggested using Wise Judge after a bottle or two of the Clear Air.

Since this was a long-distance patient, much of the diagnosis had to be left to self-evaluation. I heard after four weeks the woman was down to one inhaler application per day and that she was able to go in for acupuncture and bulk herbs on an emergency use basis, which was preferable since the acupuncturist was a two hour drive away.

Analysis: Chronic asthma usually involves the Kidney. It is often necessary to use a short-term Mahuang formula, such as Minor Blue Dragon for Cold signs, or Clear Air for Heat signs, because these will bring symptomatic relief. In modern treatment Ginseng and Gecko is all the more important, since asthma medication tends to contain steroids, and steroids tend to damage the Kidney. Weekly acupuncture would have been preferable, but it wasn't practical in this case.

Case 5

A colleague treated a forty year-old woman with chronic asthma who had used a bronchial dilator once a day for the last few years. The practitioner prescribed Power Mushrooms and Lucid Channel. Lucid Channel was selected to dry Phlegm, and Power Mushrooms was selected to tonify her immune system. In addition, Power Mushrooms contains Ganoderma, which has been successfully used to treat a variety of bronchial conditions, and herbs such as Poria which are draining. Within a month of taking one tablet of each formula per day (she was supposed to take one of each TID) she reported that she only had to take her dilator approximately once a month.

Breast Fibroids

Western Medicine

Up to fifty percent of adult women have fibrocystic disease of the breast. The cyst is tender and moves freely, whereas a cancerous growth does not usually move, and is harder. It is important for women with abnormal growths to get a medical diagnosis as soon as possible to rule out cancer. About one woman in nine in the U.S. has breast cancer in her lifetime.

TCM

Stagnation of Liver Qi, Blood, and accumulated Phlegm.

Bupleurum Entangled Qi Formula

Ingredients

English	pinyin
Bupleurum	Chai Hu
Tang-kuei	Dang Gui
Blue Citrus	Qing Pi
Prunella	Xia Ku Cao
Salvia	Dan Shen
Tricosanthes root	Tian Hua Fen
Vaccaria	Wang Bu Liu Xing
White Peony	Bai Shao
Cyperus	Xiang Fu
Ligusticum	Chuan Xiong
Fritillaria	Chuan Bei Mu
Dandelion	Pu Gong Ying
Red Peony	Chi Shao

(see also: Clear Heat)

Chinese Herbal Therapy

Bupleurum Entangled Qi Formula has produced very good results over the years. It contains herbs for activating Blood and Qi circulation, with herbs to resolve Phlegm and clear Heat and Toxin. If there is lymphatic swelling, also use Clear Heat, which contains additional herbs for clearing Heat and clearing Toxin, particularly Laminaria, which helps reduce lymphatic swelling.

Notes

Naturopathic treatment involves a low-fat diet and removal of all caffeine.

Case Study

A thirty-six year-old woman with fibrocystic breast disease had several fibroids, the largest being 5 cm (approximately two inches). After four months of using Bupleurum Entangled Qi, three tablets TID, the same fibroid was reduced in size to 0.5 cm.

Candidiasis

Western Medicine

Candida albicans is present in everyone; however, in immune-compromised individuals, the yeast can proliferate and become systemic. The major body systems most sensitive to candida are the gastrointestinal, reproductive, urinary, endocrine, nervous, and immune systems. Food and pollen allergies can also be caused by candida. The major culprit in candidiasis is the overuse of antibiotics. Anti-ulcer medication, corticosteroids, oral contraceptives, and too much sugar and alcohol can also cause candidiasis. Antifungal drugs such as Nystatin and Nizoral are often prescribed. Most of the Western herbs and nutrients are not as effective as Chinese herbal therapy, since the TCM diagnosis is more sophisticated and treatment is more broad-spectrum. For example, Damp Heat herbs and antifungals will attack yeast directly, and Spleen Qi tonics will augment the immune system to help natural suppression of the candida.

TCM

Damp Heat in the Stomach, Spleen, and Intestines, Spleen Qi deficiency.

Chinese Herbal Therapy
Systemic Candida

Treatment almost always includes Damp Heat-resolving herbs, and Spleen Qi tonics in order to tonify the immune system, and eliminate fatigue and gastrointestinal symptoms. Also, antifungal herbs are highly recommended. The Phellostatin formula contains all of the above categories of herbs and is usually taken along with Quiet Digestion for the first few weeks. Quiet Digestion eliminates both food stagnation and Dampness and helps the assimilation of the herbs in Phellostatin. It is important to realize that those who have candidiasis have very poor absorption, and therefore must integrate this formula slowly, starting with one tablet TID and increasing to three tablets TID over a two to three week period. Phellostatin therapy also produces a low rate of "die off" reactions, in which the symptoms exacerbate while the yeast is dying off; fewer than 1% of patients taking Phellostatin experience such reactions. The incidence of die-off reactions in those taking Nystatin or Caprylic acid is much more common (20-30%). Patients with severe candida can take Nystatin and Phellostatin together since patients on Nystatin often notice that after Nystatin is withdrawn symptoms can increase in a rebound effect. It is recommended that antifungal herbs not be administered in tea form because the absorption is too quick.

Vaginal Candida

For vaginal candida (i.e. "yeast infection") use Vagistatin as a vaginal insert, one or two capsules each night until the condition is cleared.

Notes

Eliminating alcohol, sugar, and yeast-containing foods is considered essential. In a strict antifungal diet, the patient eats nothing but meat and vegetables because everything else may contain or feed the yeast. After a period of time it may be possible to reintroduce and evaluate yeast-containing foods; however, the alcohol and sugar must still be avoided. The TCM diet with the above-mentioned modifications is extremely important.

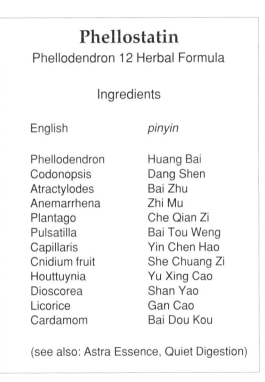

Phellostatin
Phellodendron 12 Herbal Formula

Ingredients

English	*pinyin*
Phellodendron	Huang Bai
Codonopsis	Dang Shen
Atractylodes	Bai Zhu
Anemarrhena	Zhi Mu
Plantago	Che Qian Zi
Pulsatilla	Bai Tou Weng
Capillaris	Yin Chen Hao
Cnidium fruit	She Chuang Zi
Houttuynia	Yu Xing Cao
Dioscorea	Shan Yao
Licorice	Gan Cao
Cardamom	Bai Dou Kou

(see also: Astra Essence, Quiet Digestion)

Astra Essence has been an excellent adjunct to Phellostatin in order to tonify the immune system and Kidney. It can improve the effectiveness of Phellostatin.

Case Studies
Case 1

A practitioner called to say that the Minor Blue Dragon formula was not producing any results for her fifty-two year-old patient with candidiasis and chronic sinus problems. The woman usually had clear phlegm, which was the reason Minor Blue Dragon was recommended.

I have found treating the Spleen to be productive for sinus problems, along with treating the sinus symptoms. I suggested using Xanthium Relieve Surface three tablets TID. Because she frequently got sinus infections that were treated with antibiotics, and also had candida, with occasional green phlegm, I suggested she take Isatis Gold. This formula, in addition to being a natural antibiotic, also resolves Phlegm, and helps reduce candida, although the latter was not a primary reason for using this formula. Isatis Gold was taken two tablets TID. After the first bottle, I suggested using Quiet Digestion instead of the Isatis Gold, and following up with the Phellostatin formula for several months. Other formulas such as the Six Gentlemen are often used to tonify the Spleen if the patient does not have candidiasis.

Case 2

A female patient in her mid-thirties was put on Nystatin by her medical doctor for her systemic candidiasis. After several weeks she was taken off Nystatin and her candida count was three times as high as it had been before going on Nystatin.

Her acupuncturist put her on Phellostatin, Acidophilus and Bifidus. after two months the patient's candida count was reduced fifty percent.

Some physicians combine Phellostatin with Nystatin since the rebound effect described above is common with antifungal drugs. Phellostatin works better in association with Acidophilus and Bifidus than by itself. Good probiotic products must be kept refrigerated.

Case 3: Vaginal Candidiasis

A nineteen year-old woman with a vaginal yeast infection took two capsules of Vagistatin vaginally before bedtime. The condition was gone the next day.

Cervical Dysplasia (Abnormal Pap)
Genital Warts

Western Medicine

Cervical dysplasia is an abnormal cellular condition within the cervix, and is generally regarded as a precancerous lesion. Class I is the least severe; Class V cervical dysplasia is considered Carcinoma *in situ.* It is believed that Herpes Simplex II and the Human Papilloma Virus (HPV) play contributing roles toward cervical dysplasia. Genital warts are caused by the HPV virus. According to Planned Parenthood, more than 40% of the U.S. population is infected with HPV. Only 2-3% of that population has a lesion that is visible to the naked eye. Vinegar and magnification, Pap smears, and DNA probes can also detect HPV, although the first and third diagnostic methods are rarely used. Other risk factors of cervical dysplasia include early age of first intercourse, multiple sex partners, smoking, oral contraception use, and nutritional deficiencies, including beta-carotene, folic acid, vitamin B6, and vitamin C.

Those with Class I-III dysplasia should get regular gynecological exams, and can try nutritional and herbal therapy. Class IV and V should get medical treatment.

TCM

Toxic Heat, Blood stagnation.

Chinese Herbal Therapy

Vagistatin is a specific formula developed by Dr. Jake Fratkin for cervical dysplasia, vaginal candidiasis, HPV, and vaginal parasites. This formula is administered vaginally in capsule form. It is based on a bulk herb prescription that was successfully used in Dr. Fratkin's clinic for many years. The decoction administration of this formula proved to be cumbersome, and so it was converted to capsules. Freeze dried yogurt has been added to the formula to help restore healthy vaginal flora. Vagistatin should be taken, along with an appropriate oral formula, for several months if it is to be used for cervical dysplasia.

A study is underway using Vagistatin, acupuncture, and dietary therapy with women with Class II cervical dysplasia.

Vagistatin
Yogurt Acidophilus Herbal Formula

Ingredients

English	*pinyin*
Isatis extract	Ban Lan Gen and Da Qing Ye
Phellodendron	Huang Bai
Salvia	Dan Shen
Artemisia	Qing Hao
Houttuynia	Yu Xing Cao
Cnidium fruit	She Chuang Zi
Agrimony	Xian He Cao

Non-fat yogurt cultured with 5.0×10^7 flora/gram; L. acidophilus, L. yogurtii, L. bulgaricus, S. thermophilus.

(see also: Unlocking, Crampbark Plus)

Unlocking is an oral formula which addresses Blood and Qi stagnation that has become bound with Damp Heat. Unlocking should be taken three tablets TID, for at least three to six months if signs and symptoms indicate. It is also indicated for endometriosis and pelvic inflammatory disease, if due to Heat.

Case Study

A practitioner in her late thirties was diagnosed with cervical dysplasia (Class II). She started taking Vagistatin, one capsule vaginally each night before bed, ate a diet with a minimum of fat and sugar, and got another Pap smear four weeks later which revealed her cervical dysplasia had returned to Class I.

This formula was based on an empirical formula that gets similar results, though usually taking more time. For example, on the same formula, a woman with Class III cervical dysplasia took six months to return to Class I.

Chemical Exposure, Environmental Sensitivity, EMS

Western Medicine

Air pollution, paint, hair sprays, household cleaning supplies, petroleum products, and insecticides are some of the substances that can cause chemical allergies. Mercury in dental fillings can cause heavy metal toxicity. People who work around toxic chemicals, or who use chemical sprays in excess may become poisoned. Lead poisoning is a concern due to old peeling lead-based paint and to emissions of lead accumulated in the soil from leaded gasoline. Lead from water piping, from seals on canned foods, and from glazing of ceramic products can also leach into food. Artists and hobbyists may unknowingly handle toxic materials on a regular basis.

It is important to find out what chemical substance has caused an allergic reaction and to stay away from those substances. Patients who have been chemically exposed should find an allergy specialist.

Patients sensitive to chemicals may be exposed to the same quantities of toxins as other people, but for unknown reasons, possibly a dysfunctional immune system, they are unable to function around an offending agent or agents.

Eosinophilia Myalgia Syndrome (EMS) is a particular disease caused not by tryptophan, as is assumed, but due to a manufacturing defect by one Japanese manufacturer of this amino acid.

TCM

TCM strategy is to protect and repair the liver by tonifying Yin and Blood. Repeated Toxic exposure may also create Liver Heat or Liver Fire. Since the skin is an organ of elimination, some patients may develop skin reactions as a result of acupuncture and herbs, as the toxins do not leave via the urine or feces.

Chinese Herbal Therapy

Ecliptex contains herbs that protect liver function and repair liver damage. This formula contains milk thistle (Silybum), which is the most frequently used Western liver-protective herb. Eclipta (Han Lian Cao) is said to even be more protective than milk thistle. The remaining herbs all have liver-protectant and/or regenerative effects according to laboratory research conducted in China and Europe. This formula should be used for at least six months.

Coptis Purge Fire may be used with Liver Heat or Liver Fire, with caution. Individuals with chemical sensitivity may need to be started on a digestive such as Quiet Digestion before tonic herbs are started. Astra Isatis may be used with Heat signs because this detoxifies the Liver with Bupleurum (Chai Hu) and has other Heat-clearing herbs and immune-enhancing ingredients. Astra Essence may also be used to tonify the Kidney Yin and Yang.

Ecliptex
Liver Protection Formula

Ingredients

English	Latin/*pinyin*
Eclipta Concentrate	Han Lian Cao
Milk Thistle (Silybum)	Silybum marianum
Curcuma	Yu Jin
Salvia	Dan Shen
Lycium Fruit	Gou Qi Zi
Ligustrum	Nu Zhen Zi
Bupleurum	Chai Hu
Schizandra	Wu Wei Zi
Tienchi Ginseng	San Qi
Tang-kuei	Dang Gui
Plantago Seed	Che Qian Zi
Licorice	Gan Cao

(see also: Coptis Purge Fire, Astra Isatis, Astra Essence, Bioradiance)

Case Studies

Case 1: Herbal Sensitivity

A woman in her late twenties was seen by her acupuncturist for an oral herpes blister that was not going away despite taking L-lysine and other supplements. The acupuncturist treated her with acupuncture and administered two different formulas to clear Heat from the Liver. One day after administering the second formula she began to break out in a rash that lasted two weeks. It turned out this patient worked with lead on a daily basis, and had several emotional stressors in her life. In addition, she was consuming L-lysine which has warming properties, and obviously herpes contributed to the Heat. Therefore the herbs and acupuncture accomplished the desired goal of getting the toxins to leave the body, however they did so via the skin rather than through the urine or stools, as would have been more desired. The conclusion I have gained is to be very careful when treating patients with toxic exposure.

Case 2: Herbal Sensitivity

A practitioner called up and said that Stomach Tabs made a patient feel like she had high blood pressure. Was there an alternate formula she could use? My first thought was that this was impossible, and I thought the patient must have been doing something like eating spicy foods. Even Ayurvedic herbs could have been causing the symptoms since Ayurveda often uses herbs that warm up the stomach, for digestive disorders.

Stomach Tabs does however contain Bupleurum. Bupleurum boosts the Yang Qi and could give the patient the feeling of Heat rising, which would feel like high blood pressure. I suggested the practitioner evaluate formulas such as Quiet Digestion, which reduces Dampness and food stagnation or Heavenly Water, which helps reduce Liver Qi stagnation and also dries Dampness.

Case 3: Environmental Illness/Chemical Exposure

A woman in her mid-thirties, who was diagnosed as environmentally ill, had been living in total seclusion for the past year. She had been eating nothing but bread and milk, and was terrified by life in general. She was referred to me by a colleague practicing hypnosis and spiritual counseling. This woman had a distended stomach, emaciated appearance, and a meek demeanor. I recommended one half of one tablet of Quiet Digestion (they break apart easily) daily with meals. She was encouraged to eat a more nutritious diet, introducing white rice and cooked vegetables first.

After three weeks she was up to one tablet of Quiet Digestion with each meal. She was encouraged to start walking every day, and live her life with health rather than sickness in mind.

After three months she was up to two tablets TID with meals, was starting to work out on a gradual basis, and had changed her living situation. Her constipation had improved, due to increased fiber and the Quiet Digestion.

After one year she was working out on a regular basis, had begun a relationship, and was looking for work. She no longer had the distended stomach or emaciated appearance, and possessed a healthy glow.

Analysis: Although hypnosis and spiritual healing played a big part in her success, the biggest factor was her own desire to see her life differently. I put her on Quiet Digestion because I was afraid she wouldn't be able to tolerate anything else. Due to her distended stomach, and milk and bread diet, it was clear there was Dampness.

I recommend Quiet Digestion, starting with half a tablet once or twice daily, for environmentally ill patients, then gradually build up the dosage. Based on my experience with highly allergic patients, normal TCM workups are not effective since the patients are almost always allergic to the herbs.

My hypothesis is that depression and allergies are linked to Dampness, and that the body must be rid of Dampness before the system can heal. Once the body no longer has Dampness, Kidney and/or Spleen tonics may be tried, since Dampness leads to these organ deficiencies. Astra Essence and Six Gentlemen are good ways to begin; Astra Essence is a balanced Kidney tonic and Six Gentlemen tonifies the Spleen and rids the body of Dampness.

Case 4: Tryptophan-induced EMS/Chemical Exposure

A male patient in his late forties contracted EMS (Eosinophilia Myalgia Syndrome) due to tainted tryptophan from a particular Japanese supplier. (There is no evidence that there is a problem with tryptophan itself.) The patient was emaciated, and his skin lacked lustre. He had lost thirty pounds since contracting the disease and had no energy. Previously he had run several miles per day and he had a busy professional practice. He had decided to try Chinese herbs as a last resort.

I suggested Bioradiance, an extremely strong extract of Chinese and Western herbs, three drops BID on a cracker, with meals. The third week, four to six drops TID on a cracker with meals, along with Astra Isatis and Power Mushrooms, two tablets of each TID. The Bioradiance was administered to knock out the infection, the other formulas were administered to counter the cooling effects of Bioradiance, and to tonify the immune system.

Three months later the patient reported that due to my recommendations, and pure tryptophan (an antidote), his life was saved. He regained most of his weight and was starting to jog lightly in the morning. Since he was having difficult breathing, with signs of Heat, I put him on Clear Air, and continued with Astra Isatis to attack the latent virus. I suggested after another month to switch to Astra Essence since he had been on Astra Isatis for several months.

Chemotherapy and Radiotherapy

Western Medicine

Side effects of chemotherapy include hair loss, extreme nausea, vomiting, fatigue, weakness, sterility, and damage to the kidneys and heart.

TCM

Chemotherapy and radiation therapy can cause rising Heat, Kidney Yin deficiency, Kidney Yang deficiency, Blood deficiency, Blood stagnation, and Spleen deficiency.

Chinese Herbal Therapy

Tableted herbs are very successful in these cases, as the patients often cannot tolerate raw herbs. Quiet Digestion effectively treats nausea, and Astra Essence is a good general formula as it treats Kidney Yin dehciency, Yang deficiency, and Blood deficiency. Astra 8 can be used if there is weak Spleen and Lung Qi, and Clear Heat has been successfully used with rising Heat. Marrow Plus is useful for bone marrow suppression, which is almost always a factor. Power Mushrooms is used for enhancing the immune system; it is not recommended if there is a lot of Heat. Master Herbalist Fung Fung uses a formula called Regeneration which contains herbs with blood circulating and other properties.

Case Studies

Case 1

A man in his late fifties was given Marrow Plus and Power Mushrooms five weeks prior to chemotherapy in order to help his body prepare. He reported greater energy level two weeks after taking the herbs. Upon beginning chemotherapy he started to show Heat signs, and was switched to Clear Heat. He took two tablets of Marrow Plus, one tablet of Astra Essence, and two tablets of Clear Heat TID. He also took Quiet Digestion as needed. The nurses and doctors were happy that he did not have to miss any chemotherapy.

Case 2

Another male patient in his late fifties with both lung cancer and pancreatic cancer responded very well, in terms of general well-being, to Power Mushrooms and Marrow Plus, two tablets of each TID, begun four weeks before chemotherapy. These tonic herbs strengthen the Blood and Qi, helping the body prepare for chemotherapy. Upon starting chemotherapy the patient began developing Heat signs and I suggested adding Clear Heat. I also suggested replacing Power Mushrooms with Astra Essence to help tonify the Kidney. He was then taking 2 tablets of Astra Essence, 2 tablets of Clear Heat, and 1 tablet of Marrow Plus TID. Power Mushrooms, although beneficial to the immune system, can cause an exacerbation of Heat signs. The strategy of treatment here is to lessen the severity of side effects to the chemotherapy.

Marrow Plus

Milletia Herbal Formula

Ingredients

English	pinyin
Milletia	Ji Xue Teng
Ho-shou-wu	He Shou Wu
Salvia	Dan Shen
Codonopsis	Dang Shen
Astragalus	Huang Qi
Ligusticum	Chuan Xiong
Raw Rehmannia	Sheng Di Huang
Cooked Rehmannia	Shu Di Huang
Lycium	Gou Ji Zi
Tang-kuei	Dang Gui
Lotus Seed	Lian Zi
Citrus	Chen Pi
Red Date Extract	Da Zao
Oryza	Gu Ya
Gelatinum	E Jiao

(see also: Astra 8, Backbone, Eight Treasures)

Case 3

A colleague had good results with a woman during chemotherapy. Using both Astra Essence and Marrow Plus, the patient's white cells increased, and she had better energy. The oncologist was pleased, and increased her chemotherapy dosage.

Case 4

A fifty-three year-old woman who had received radiation for breast cancer developed hot flashes and was taking anti-estrogenic therapy. The practitioner wondered if she could use Two Immortals.

Two Immortals has been used with success in cases of radiotherapy for breast cancer. Radiation often causes Toxic Heat, and can also cause Kidney Yin and Yang deflciency. Therefore I suggested using three tablets TID of Two Immortals, which supplements Kidney Yin and Yang, with one or more tablets of Clear Heat TID. Based on my experience, the patient should start feeling better in about two weeks, if she is taking the recommended dosage.

Case 5

A fifty year-old woman with liver cancer, who previously had breast cancer, was undergoing chemotherapy and due to start radiation in a few weeks. The patient had a lot of pain and was taking morphine prescribed by her medical doctor. This woman had signs of Heat and Blood stagnation.

I suggested a combination of Clear Heat, which has proved very useful as an adjunct formula for chemo- and radiotherapy; Marrow Plus, which activates and tonifies Blood, and is also useful for the side effects of chemo- and radiotherapy; and Astra Essence, which tonifies Essence (Jing), Yin, and Yang. Recommended dosage was two tablets each of the three formulas TID. If the patient had any digestive problems, Quiet Digestion would have been added. This combination of formulas treats the indicated TCM signs and supports the Kidney.

Case 6

A patient came to our clinic with Lung Cancer and other complications due to having one kidney removed. The patient had also gone through chemo and radiotherapy and was very weak. He was recommended to take bulk herbs as well as Regeneration. After six months western tests revealed no further cancer growth. The patient feels more energetic since taking the herbs.

Case 7

Another patient on chemotherapy reported her nausea stopped one day after taking Quiet Digestion.

Chronic Fatigue Immune Dysfunction Syndrome (CFIDS)

Western Medicine

Chronic Fatigue Immune Dysfunction Syndrome (CFIDS) may include chronic fatigue, low grade fever, lymphatic swelling, headache, muscle and joint pain, recurrent sore throats, digestive disorders, depression, and loss of concentration. Researchers believe that CFIDS may be caused by Epstein-Barr virus, other viruses or virus combinations that cause or are caused by immune dysfunction, *Candida albicans* fungus, anemia, chronic mercury poisoning from amalgam fillings, hypoglycemia, or hypothyroidism. You should rule out Lyme Disease, AIDS, infections, anemia, and parasites which can cause similar symptoms. Antidepressants are sometimes prescribed.

TCM

Spleen Qi deficiency, Kidney Yin and Yang deficiency, Toxic Heat, Spleen Dampness, Stagnant Liver Qi.

Chinese Herbal Therapy

(See also the appendix: Treating CFIDS in the Clinic.)

Successful TCM treatment depends upon diagnosis. My first approach is to make sure there is no Dampness and therefore the digestive system is functioning correctly. Therefore the first formula may be Quiet Digestion. If there are particular problems with digesting meals, recommend Quiet Digestion one tablet before and one tablet after meals. Two formulas that have been successfully used are Astra Isatis and Power Mushrooms. Astra Isatis is taken three tablets TID, and Power Mushrooms is usually started at two tablets per day. This combination of formulas addresses Spleen Qi deficiency, Kidney Yin and Yang deficiency, lymphatic swelling, and Liver stagnation, and tonifies the immune system. If there are Heat signs, or high levels of viral activity, use Astra Isatis with Clear Heat. Patients with Cold signs will do better with Astra 8 and Power Mushrooms. Patients may also take Astra 8 and Astra Isatis simultaneously. Ecliptex may be appropriate, particularly if there are high liver SGOT enzymes and Liver Qi stagnation. Nine Flavor Tea is used if there is Yin deficiency. Thus adjunct formulas are used in addition to Astra Isatis. If there are signs of deficient Blood and Blood stagnation, Enhance may be used. It is suggested that patients take these protocols for two to three months and then alternate the base formula. Thus if the patient has taken Astra Isatis for three months, have them take Enhance for one month before resuming Astra Isatis.

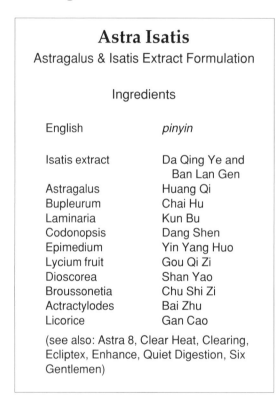

Astra Isatis
Astragalus & Isatis Extract Formulation

Ingredients

English	pinyin
Isatis extract	Da Qing Ye and Ban Lan Gen
Astragalus	Huang Qi
Bupleurum	Chai Hu
Laminaria	Kun Bu
Codonopsis	Dang Shen
Epimedium	Yin Yang Huo
Lycium fruit	Gou Qi Zi
Dioscorea	Shan Yao
Broussonetia	Chu Shi Zi
Actractylodes	Bai Zhu
Licorice	Gan Cao

(see also: Astra 8, Clear Heat, Clearing, Ecliptex, Enhance, Quiet Digestion, Six Gentlemen)

CFIDS patients may get frequent viral or bacterial infections. If this is the case, use three tablets Isatis Gold every few hours and discontinue the other more tonifying herbs until symptoms abate (see Colds & Flu).

Notes
Recommend eating cooked food only, following TCM diet, and getting light exercise.

Case Studies
Case 1
A twenty-four year-old woman diagnosed with CFIDS was suffering from shooting pains throughout her body, fevers that would rise suddenly and then fall quickly, night sweats, painful and swollen lymph nodes, bleeding cracks in the mouth, alternating constipation and diarrhea, asthma, allergies, occasional cognitive difficulties, persistent infections, shooting and distending pain in her right abdomen, hypochondria, extreme fatigue, and other symptoms.

She was bedridden and had tried Zovirax, without improvement. An acupuncturist treated her with acupuncture and various herbal formulas, which she eventually learned to take herself, with help from her practitioner, since her symptoms where always changing. The base program was Astra Isatis, which contains immune-enhancing and antiviral herbs (according to research conducted in China), and Ecliptex, which contains herbs such as Milk Thistle *(Silybum marianum)* and Eclipta (Han Lian Cao) which have liver-protectant and liver-regenerative effects (according to laboratory research carried out in Europe and China). She also took Astra 8, which strengthens Lung, Spleen, and general immunity. Other formulas were used as well to strengthen immunity, tonify Yin and Yang, and reduce Toxic Heat.

After slowly regaining her health, five years later she began to run, and now six years later she has won five-kilometer races, and has a chance to make it as a professional duathlon athlete. She continues to use herbs as needed.

Analysis: This was a severe case, and no single formula cured this patient's Chronic Fatigue. It was a combination of acupuncture and the correct herbal formula for each changing set of conditions. Since the changing patterns in chronic disorders are often consistent, practitioners can instruct patients to use formulas for the specific patterns on their own. Patients always have to keep in mind the larger goal, and remember reasons to get well. If there are no strong reasons, the body and mind would just as soon stay sick, since that is what the body and mind are used to.

Case 2

A patient in his early forties had multiple allergies and at one time had been treated for parasites and chronic fatigue. The patient looked tired and had facial flushing. He said he could not take bulk herbs because they make him sick. The patient had a fast pulse and deficient-looking tongue. His practitioner recommended Bu Zhong Yi Qi Tang (Arouse Vigor), which he took, and it made him sick. I suspected Spleen Dampness and told him to take Quiet Digestion right before meals. I also recommended Clearing, as Clearing treats loose stools, and contains Yin tonics without Rehmannia. Patients with digestive problems often cannot digest Rehmannia, and occasionally not Astragalus. Bu Zhong Yi Qi Tang made the patient feel worse, which indicated that this patient's deficient feeling was due mostly to Damp Heat. After one day the patient remarked that Quiet Digestion was the best formula he had tried in years.

The patient was anxious to try something for energy, so I recommended Astra Essence, which he was unable to digest. He found Six Gentlemen helpful. One month later he had remarkably better energy, and was told to remain on the Quiet Digestion, Clearing, and Six Gentlemen protocol for a few more months to clear up the chronic Dampness.

Case 3

A forty-four year-old man, medically diagnosed with Epstein-Barr virus, was put on Enhance by his practitioner. Some improvement was noted, however the patient continued to have sore throats, therefore the practitioner called me. I suggested that he discontinue Enhance and treat the patient with Nine Flavor Tea, since the majority of his symptoms, including the sore throat, were indicative of a Yin deficiency pattern. His tongue was red and dry.

The patient's chronic sore throat went away, but his medical doctor put him on antibiotics for an unknown reason and the sore throat came back. The practitioner was concerned about mixing herbs and antibiotics.

I replied that there usually is not a problem with combining herbs and antibiotics. It is my personal opinion that antibiotics cause Dampness. I suggested that the practitioner continue using the Nine Flavor Tea, since the patient had a healthy digestive system. If the patient had a weak digestive system I would suggest adding Quiet Digestion, since Rehmannia (Shu Di Huang) and other Yin tonics may cause Dampness if administered over a long period, or with patients who have weak digestive systems.

Unfortunately this was a difficult patient because he would feel better, go skiing for a few days, and then feel totally wiped out, and then would go skiing again once he began to feel better. I also suggested that he think of his health like a bank account, to be deposited into instead of constantly spent.

Case 4

A housebound woman in her late thirties, diagnosed with CFIDS as well as malabsorption, reported fatigue, insomnia, loose stools, anxiety, headaches, gas, bloating, stomach growling, loss of appetite, and burning in the stomach. She had a thin rapid pulse, and her tongue was red, dry, and had a yellow coat in the center. She was taking anti-anxiety medication, Gather Vitality (Gui Pi Tang), and Schizandra Dreams, which helped her insomnia.

I suggested she not take Gather Vitality at the present time since it didn't seem that she could digest the Blood tonic and Qi tonic herbs contained in this herbal formula. It is always my practice to clear up the digestive problems before adding tonic herbs. Therefore, I suggested she take one tablet of Quiet Digestion every two hours, and take Stomach Tabs, two tablets TID.

After two weeks I had her discontinue the Stomach Tabs and take Clearing, three tablets, TID, with one tablet of Quiet Digestion before and after meals. Although her digestion had improved, her main signs were Heat signs, I believe due to the anti-anxiety medication. Clearing contains Heat-clearing herbs, and also treats Dampness. The patient continued taking Schizandra Dreams before bed or as needed throughout the day. Since this formula contains Dragonbone (Long Gu) and Oystershell (Mu Li) it is able to bring down rising Liver Yang. I did not use Coptis Purge Fire (based on Long Dan Xie Gan Tang with additional herbs) because I was afraid it would be too draining for this patient.

Four weeks after beginning the herbs, the patient's digestive problems were greatly improved as were her loose stools. She said she felt "more together" than she had in along time, which I felt was a result of resolving some of the Dampness. Her tongue did not have a yellow coat, although it was dry and red. Her fatigue was lessened, although many of the other symptoms remained. At this point I added Calm Spirit, two tablets TID, to give her additional Heart stabilizing and Yin tonification.

She is pleased with our results and she continues to use herbs, acupuncture, and psychotherapy.

Case 5

A woman in her late thirties, with a CFIDS diagnosis for the past five years, was unable to work. She had constant severe headaches for which the medical doctors prescribed Vicadin, which contains a semi-synthetic narcotic analgesic. She also suffered from fatigue, depression, nausea, indigestion, and low grade afternoon fevers, and reported that Compound GL and Astra 8 produced no effect.

On careful examination it appeared that this patient belonged to the Yin deficient type of CFIDS. Her tongue was red and dry, her left pulse was deep and fast on the left side, on the right side a pulse couldn't be found.

I suggested using Gastrodia Relieve Wind, as I believe Yin deficiency is brought about Internal Wind. In addition I have had good success using this formula with difficult cases. Perhaps there is more Internal Wind than we realize in America. This formula was recommended, with Fertile Garden, to supplement Yin without cooked Rehmannia, and with Quiet Digestion taken before and after meals to help her assimilate food.

The practitioner I was working with asked how long she should try these herbs before giving up, since past herbal formulas had no effect. I said a month at the full dosage, taking two tablets of each formula TID. Housebound patients often say they can't take this many pills. I pointed out if the patient took less than this dosage, it would take longer to get results.

Case 6

A colleague was treating a successful businessman who was diagnosed as having mononucleosis. The practitioner put him on Power Mushrooms and Astra Isatis. After one month he wasn't getting any better. After inquiry, I found that he was only taking one tablet of each formula per day because he was taking so many other things: blue-green algae, a multivitamin, vitamin C, garlic capsules, echinacea, as well as catnip and other supplements he picked up at a health food store.

He was reinstructed to take three Astra Isatis TID, one tablet of Power Mushroom TID, continue the multivitamin, and stop taking everything else until he was healthy. Two months after using the formulas at the correct dosage level, he was able to play basketball and resume his normal schedule.

Analysis: The problem with self-treatment is that unless people get quick results they often keep adding supplement after supplement without taking adequate quantities of anything. Unfortunately, this is extremely common.

Case 7

A male client in his forties with a previous history of herpes zoster complained of fatigue so severe that he could only work two or three days per week. He had afternoon malaise and facial flushing, chronic sinusitis with feelings of being stuffed up all the time and with no drainage, gastric upset when he ate grains, and occasional episodes of severe arthritis whereby all joints, particularly ones he used frequently, throbbed and ached with no swelling. He also reported multiple allergies, especially to molds and mildews, and frequent colds and flus. His tongue had a crack down the middle but was normal colored. His pulse was deficient. Western medical doctors had ruled out AIDS, Lupus, and MS. The client reported that an echinacea and ganoderma (reishi) product from the health food store made him feel too stimulated.

The patient was put on Mobility 2 for an acute arthritis attack. He got considerable relief taking three tablets TID. Follow-up therapy involved using Astra Isatis, three tablets TID, to attack latent virus and to tonify his Spleen Qi, Kidney Yin and Kidney Yang. I also suggested taking Astra C, one tablet TID to tonify his Wei Qi, dry Dampness, and boost his immunity, since Astra C contains vitamin C and zinc.

After six weeks the client reported steady improvement. He likes taking the herbs especially in the afternoon, as they lessen his malaise.

Circulatory Disorders, Angina, Intermittent Claudication, Mental Deterioration

Western Medicine

Many circulatory disorders are recognized in Western medicine. Arteriosclerosis or "hardening of the arteries" is due to cholesterol as well as narrowing of the arteries. Circulatory problems may lead to angina or stroke. Chronic inflammation of the veins and arteries in the lower parts of the body is Buerger's disease. Raynaud's syndrome is characterized by constriction and spasm of the blood vessels in the extremities.

Complications due to atherosclerosis are the leading causes of death in the U.S. The arteries degenerate due to a build-up of cholesterol and other lipids within the arteries. An initial lesion in the arterial wall may be necessary before the lipids can accumulate. Standard medical therapy may involve a low-fat diet, nitroglycerine, beta channel blockers, coronary balloon angioplasty, and bypass surgery.

TCM

Blood stagnation, Phlegm obstruction, Yin deficiency, Qi deficiency, Blood deficiency.

Chinese Herbal Therapy

Flavonex is an excellent formula for all patients with circulatory disorders. It should be given for more than a year, and the dosage is three tablets TID.

For intermittent claudication, Flavonex can be combined with Cir-Q. If the patient has obvious Cold signs, add two tablets of Cir-Q BID. This formula will also be effective if there is a chronic Cold Damp condition. If the patient has obvious Heat signs do not use Cir-Q or else use it cautiously. This protocol may also be used for patients with varicose veins.

If there are palpitations, anxiety, insomnia, pale complexion, pale lips, poor memory, with a pale tongue, this may be Heart Blood deficiency; Shen-Gem may be added to Flavonex. This formula is based on Gui Pi Tang (Ginseng and Longan Formula).

Oftentimes, long-standing use of pharmaceutical drugs may cause Yin deficiency. If there is feeling of Heat particularly in the evening, dry mouth and throat, malar flush, and red peeled tongue, Calm Spirit (based on Ding Xin Wan) is an excellent adjunct to Flavonex.

If there are signs of Heart Yin deficiency, characterized by palpitations, insomnia, poor memory, anxiety, low grade fever, feeling of heat in the evening, night sweating, dry mouth, warm extremities, and mental restlessness, the patient should take

Flavonex	
Salvia and Ginkgo Extract Formulation	
Ingredients	
English	*pinyin*
Pueraria	Ge Gen
Ilex	Mao Dong Qing
Salvia	Dan Shen
Lonicera	Jin Yin Hua
Eucommia	Du Zhong
Acorus	Shi Chang Pu
Cistanche	Rou Cong Rong
Ho-shou-wu	He Shou Wu
Morus fruit	Sang Ren
Rosa	Jin Ying Zi
Lycium fruit	Gou Qi Zi
Zizyphus	Suan Zao Ren
Tang-kuei	Dang Gui
Schizandra	Wu Wei Zi
Ginkgo biloba extract	Bai Guo Ye

(see also: Cir-Q, Shen Gem, Gather Vitality, Calm Spirit)

Calm Spirit. A more severe condition is Heart Fire Blazing, characterized by mouth ulcers, agitation, feeling of heat, insomnia, red face, dark urine or blood in the urine, red tongue with swollen tip and yellow coating, rapid pulse, thirst and palpitations. Use Coptis Purge Fire (based on Long Dan Xie Gan Tang) with Schizandra Dreams.

Successful treatment works hand in hand with Western diagnosis and treatment, and is based on TCM diagnosis. Cir-Q was developed on the basis of a Tibetan remedy used in Switzerland that activates blood circulation, resolves Phlegm, and regulates Qi. Many of these herbs work best in tablet form, because the aromatic components evaporate with boiling. It is a warming formula and must be used sparingly with Yin deficient patients, or else modified with a Yin tonic. It will be effective for patients suffering from angina or intermittent claudication.

Flavonex contains Ginkgo leaf extract, which has been proven to increase circulation in several double blind studies. It combines Chinese herbs such as Pueraria (Ge Gen), Ilex (Mao Dong Qing), Salvia (Dan Shen), Ho shou wu, and Tang-kuei, which have been proven to increase circulation and microcirculation, with other bioflavonoid herbs that strengthen the capillaries and reduce inflammation. Therefore Flavonex, which is balanced so it isn't too warming or too cooling, can be added to Cir-Q if there is obstruction with Cold symptoms, to Calm Spirit if there are Heat signs, or to Gastrodia Relieve Wind if there are signs of high blood pressure or Internal Wind (see High Blood Pressure).

Cir-Q
Aromatic Herbal Compound

Ingredients

English	*pinyin*
Cardamon	Bai Dou Kou
Eucommia	Du Zhong
Sandalwood	Tan Xiang
Saussurea	Mu Xiang
Borneol	Bing Pian
Melia	Chuan Lian Zi
Myrobalan	He Zi
Aquilaria	Chen Xiang
Prunella	Xia Ku Cao
Aristolochia	Ma Dou Ling
Cloves	Ding Xiang
Hardy Orange	Zhi Shi
Ginger	Gan Jiang
Licorice	Gan Cao
Frankincense	Ru Xiang
Acorus	Shi Chang Pu

(see also: Calm Spirit, Flavonex, Gastrodia Relieve Wind)

Notes

Patients should stop smoking and drinking alcohol and coffee, adopt a TCM diet, engage in a stress reduction program, and exercise daily. Many nutrients including CO-Q-10, EPA, vitamin E, and carnitine may be helpful.

Case Study

A woman in her late fifties, with a biomedical diagnosis of arteritis and symptoms of Raynaud's syndrome, was taking prednisone with calcium supplementation. I suggested adding magnesium in a proportion of one part magnesium to two parts calcium. I also recommended Flavonex, three tablets TID.

After five weeks she reported that it was much easier for her to climb hills without having to stop and catch her breath. I suggested she continue to take Flavonex for the next five years.

Colds and Flu

Western Medicine

Rest, drink plenty of liquids.

TCM

It is important to differentiate between Wind Heat and Wind Cold.

Chinese Herbal Therapy

The well-known Yin Chao is only effective for the initial stage of a Wind Heat attack. Effective Western herbs include echinacea and goldenseal. They are frequently included in Western herbal cold and flu treatments. The beauty in these herbs is that they are very effective at resolving Phlegm, and are more suitable than Yin Chao for the second or third stages of a cold or flu. They can be used with either Wind Heat or Wind Cold. They are combined with isatis extract (Da Qing Ye and Ban Lan Gen), platycodon (Jie Geng) for the Lung, and ligusticum (Chuan Xiong) to make a very effective cold and flu formula called Isatis Gold.

In a **Wind Cold** attack, characterized by chills, sneezing, coughing, runny nose with white phlegm, occipital stiffness and ache, no sweating or thirst, use Isatis Gold, three tablets every two to three hours with fresh ginger tea (1 tsp fresh ginger slices per 8 oz). If there is headache, Head-Q may be combined. Use Minor Blue Dragon if there is Lung involvement with white phlegm.

With **Wind Heat** symptoms, characterized by runny nose with yellow phlegm, fever, sweating, sore throat, swollen tonsils, thirst, red tongue coat on tip or sides, use Isatis Gold, three tablets every two to three hours. Combine with Clear Air, two tablets every few hours, if the cold or flu has entered into the lungs, and there is yellow phlegm. If there is digestive upset, Isatis Gold may be combined with Quiet Digestion.

Notes

Eating should be light, and everything eaten should be warm and easily digestible. It is important to get plenty of rest, drink lots of fluids. The Wind Cold patient should keep warm at all times. Bringing on a light sweat by drinking ginger or black tea is recommended to move out the infection in the case of Wind Cold; it is important that the patient be covered up.

Case Studies

Case 1

A client was running a slight fever, had an achy feeling all over, a barking cough, copious yellow-green phlegm, and a rapid pulse. She took a combination of Isatis Gold and Clear Air, two tablets of each every three hours. By the next day all symptoms were considerably better.

Case 2

A client had the signs of a Wind Cold invasion, slow, submerged pulse, pale tongue, little energy, headache, and coughing. I used a combination of Minor Blue Dragon, which is used for Wind Cold coughing, and Isatis Gold, which I have successfully used in cases of both Wind Heat and Wind Cold.

Isatis Gold

Goldenseal, Echinacea, Isatis Extract

Ingredients

English	Latin/*pinyin*
Echinacea	Echinacea purpurea
Chaparral	Larrea divaricata
Platycodon	Jie Geng
Goldenseal	Hydrastis canadensis
Ligusticum	Chuan Xiong
Isatis extract	Da Qing Ye and Ban Lan Gen

(see also: Clear Air, Minor Blue Dragon, Yin Chao Jin)

I also advised the client to drink hot tea and abstain from raw foods. The client was taking two tablets of each formula every three to four hours.

The condition did not change after forty-eight hours, nor was there any change in symptoms, therefore I did not think to switch the formulas. Seventy-two hours after seeing me the patient got a prescription for antibiotics, and felt better the next day.

67

In talking this case over with a colleague I came to the conclusion that this was a case of Heat masquerading as Cold. It is possible that this woman, who had taken Isatis Gold on many occasions before, had gotten immune to it, or had I selected Clear Air, which would have treated hidden Heat, or used stronger exterior relieving herbs, she could have been treated using herbs. There are some cases of bronchitis that necessitate the use of antibiotics.

Constipation

Western Medicine

Laxatives are commonly prescribed. Over-the-counter laxatives are among the most frequently-used medications. Drugs and herbs used for this purpose can cause laxative dependency. Constipation is common for those who do not eat enough fiber, drink enough fluids, or get enough exercise.

TCM

Constipation is usually caused by excess Heat. Constipation in the elderly or in women after childbirth suggests Blood deficiency. Alternating constipation and diarrhea suggests Liver Qi stagnation invading the Spleen or candida infection (see also Candidiasis).

Chinese Herbal Therapy

(See also the appendix: Chinese Herbal Treatment of Chronic Digestive Disorders.)

For the elderly, or for anyone suffering from Blood deficiency, Eight Treasures is an excellent choice. It moistens the Intestines. For constipation due to Heat, which may accompany stress, a good combination is Ease Plus and Calm Spirit. Prescribe two tablets of each TID. This will moisten the Intestines, relieve Liver Qi stagnation, and bring down excess Heat. Ease Plus contains Rhubarb (Da Huang), which is a purgative.

Aquilaria 22 is the formula of choice for constipation due to parasites. It can also be used for chronic constipation with abdominal bloating, and constipation due to Qi stagnation.

Dr. Fung's Gentle Senna is a gentle formula used to regulate water content in the body and remove heat. It can be used to treat chronic constipation, and is taken before going to bed.

Notes

A high-fiber diet successfully treats most constipation. Therefore the TCM diet with regular exercise is recommended. Drinking plenty of water is also recommended.

Case Studies

Case 1

A practitioner without much experience with herbs called about a patient who was chronically constipated and was addicted to psyllium husks from the health food store. The patient was under stress and had cold hands and feet and occasional gas. I suggested a combination of Ease Plus and Calm Spirit.

Analysis: Ease Plus treats constipation accompanying stress. I reasoned there must be Liver involvement, since constipation is almost always indicative of Heat. In this context I believed the cold hands and feet were due to stagnant Liver Qi rather than Cold. Calm Spirit was also recommended to help ease the patient's stress and to lubricate the Intestines. I suggested two tablets of each TID. This combination will relieve constipation and help the patient feel les stressed, but it may take longer to warm the hands and feet.

Gentle Senna
Dr. Fung's Senna Herbal Formula

Ingredients

English	pinyin
Microcos	Po Bu Ye
Lonicera	Jin Yin Hua
Senna	Fan Xie Ye
Prunus	Yu Li Ren
Pueraria flower	Ge Hua
Areca seed	Bing Lang

(see also: Ease Plus, Aquilaria 22, Calm Spirit)

Case 2

An overweight woman in her late thirties with a history of chronic constipation that was only partially relieved by a high fiber diet, and abdominal bloating reported remarkable results after taking one bottle of Aquilaria 22, two tablets TID.

Crohn's Disease and Ulcerative Colitis

Western Medicine

Ulcerative colitis is the inflammation of the colon. Crohn's is the chronic inflammation of a section of the digestive tract. Both diseases are characterized by malabsorption. For colitis and Crohn's, regular colonoscopy is important. Long-term antibiotics and steroids may be administered.

Vitamin B12 is an excellent supplement, as well as standard B-complex vitamins. Acidophilus supplementation is highly recommended. Bovine colostrom can be helpful, especially with loose stools.

TCM

Blood stagnation, Qi deficiency, Damp Heat, food stagnation, Kidney deficiency.

Chinese Herbal Therapy

(See also the appendix: Chinese Herbal Treatment for Chronic Digestive Disorders.)

I find that almost all Crohn's and UC patients have Damp Heat and food stagnation. Two formulas have been very useful: Isatis Cooling is used when there is blood stagnation, characterized by sharp stabbing pain with inflammation; Phellostatin is used for Damp Heat with Qi deficiency. Thus Isatis Cooling is usually administered in the acute stage, whereas Phellostatin is usually administered in the chronic maintenance stage. Quiet Digestion must be administered at first every two hours if there is gas. Once gas has subsided, it can be administered one tablet before and one tablet after each meal, to help with the absorbtion of food. Formula H can be used with rectal bleeding.

Notes

The TCM diet is a major part of the therapy. Low-fiber foods are recommended. Most Crohn's and UC patients cannot tolerate tomatoes in any form. Many also have high levels of candida or sensitivity to normal levels of candida. Other common allergies such as yeast, corn, and soy should be carefully evaluated. Consider an elimination diet. Lifestyle considerations include stress reduction, acupuncture, meditation, and exercise, being careful not to exercise to exhaustion.

Case Studies
Case 1
A fifty year-old man with Crohn's disease had been on steroids off and on for more than ten years, and he was preparing to go on steroids once more, and asked his practitioner if anything could be done to avoid steroids. The symptoms as reported to me were mainly related to deficiency: that is, cold limbs with slow deficient pulse; however the tongue was reddish purple in the middle. The patient had tremendous gas and bloating, especially after meals. The patient had four to five watery stools per day with occasional constipation.

I suggested TCM diet, Quiet Digestion before and after meals, and smaller meals more frequently throughout the day. I also suggested Isatis Cooling, three tablets TID. My original plan was after six weeks to switch to the Phellostatin formula, and then gradually introduce Astra Essence, along with Six Gentlemen for the signs of Spleen Qi deficiency. For example, after six weeks the patient might take two tablets Phellostatin and two tablets Astra Essence TID until the bottle of Phellostatin is gone, and then take two Phellostatin, two Astra Essence, and two Six Gentlemen tablets TID.

After six weeks the patient reported less diarrhea and didn't feel he needed to go on steroids. However, he was still fatigued, though his tongue looked slightly better, according to the practitioner; therefore, I

Isatis Cooling

Ingredients

English	pinyin
Isatis extract	Ban Lan Gen and Da Qing Ye
Codonopsis	Dang Shen
Oyster shell	Mu Li
Bupleurum	Chai Hu
Smilax	Tu Fu Ling
Gardenia	Zhi Zi
Moutan	Mu Dan Pi
Tang-kuei	Dang Gui
Akebia	Mu Tong
Red Peony	Chi Shao
Alisma	Ze Xie
Cyperus	Xiang Fu

(see also: Phellostatin, Quiet Digestion)

suggested a slower approach than originally recommended. I decided he should stay on the Isatis Cooling, and mix with Phellostatin, two of each TID and maintain the Quiet Digestion. Whether to add Astra Essence will be evaluated in another four weeks.

Analysis: Crohn's usually involves considerable Damp Heat in the Intestines, with food stagnation, Qi deficiency, and Kidney deficiency.

Case 2

A twenty-one year-old man with a life-long history of Crohn's disease came to me after receiving nutritional therapy, hands-on therapy, Chinese herbs and acupuncture from a man in Chinatown. He was on 7 mgs of prednisone per day. When I saw him he was also taking an anti-parasitic Western herbal formula and about twenty supplements, many of which were said to counterbalance the effects of steroids. I looked at the bag of herbs and was amazed at the lack of quality. There were also some unlabeled patent medicines he was taking.

Next I inquired into his dietary habits and found out he had given up alcohol, but was drinking milk because he had no problem with lactose. Also, he liked to go out for pizza with his friends a few days per week, and liked ice water. His tongue was purple with no coat, and his pulse was very weak.

The first thing I did was tell him to stop drinking iced drinks, which are damaging to the Spleen. Second, I suggested a warm food diet, and the elimination of milk, even though he wasn't lactose intolerant, because in TCM it is considered mucous-forming. Third, I substituted Artestatin for the Western herbal anti-parasitic, which did not seem to be well-formulated. I also suggested taking Quiet Digestion, one tablet before and one after each meal, and two tablets before and after "cheating," i.e. after eating pizza, which he said contributed to nasal discharge but not to his Crohn's. Finally I suggested taking the Isatis Cooling formula along with the Artestatin, three tablets of each TID, and slowly cutting down his prednisone by 0.5 mg or 1 mg. at a time, under the supervision of his doctor. The patient was unavailable for follow-up.

Case 3

A thirty-six year-old man with Crohn's was seen by a colleague. At the time he came in he was on 20 mg of prednisone per day. After a course of Isatis Cooling and Six Gentlemen, the patient was able to drop his prednisone dosage to 11 mg per day. The condition was stable, and then one day he woke up with severe bleeding and cramping. A week before, he had come down with flu-like symptoms. The practitioner asked for my feedback and suggestions.

First of all, this type of reaction is not uncommon. One patient, after taking Isatis Cooling for seven days, reported miraculous results and then had a major setback. We added Quiet Digestion to his regimen, and he was able to eat a wider variety of foods; however, he continued to have occasional bouts of pain. Thanks to acupuncture and massage, these bouts decreased in frequency.

Analysis: In most cases we are able to control, not cure, Inflammatory Bowel Disease. Stress, and/or dietary factors can still trigger an episode at any time. If this patient had a parasitic infection, this could have caused the flu symptoms and triggered IBD symptoms; therefore, parasitic infection should be ruled out. If he caught the flu, however, only the flu symptoms should be addressed. Steroids might have been withdrawn too quickly. Finally, as with any chronic disease, Wei Qi can be particularly low, therefore formulas that increase Wei Qi, such as Astra C, and Royal Jelly, as well as internal exercises should be applied to increase resistance.

Case 4

Another case I was asked about concerned a nineteen year-old who was diagnosed with Crohn's. He had been on prescription analgesics, had gotten excellent symptomatic relief with the Quiet Digestion formula, and was experiencing swelling in the joints. His sister, who was seventeen years old, was experiencing Crohn's symptoms. I strongly urged the family members to get tested for parasites. My experience is that it is rare for siblings to have Crohn's disease.

Case 5

A rock and roll star had chronic colitis, with no pain and a lot of gas. I recommended Quiet Digestion before meals and Phellostatin at one tablet TID between meals, increased to three tablets TID over a two week period. The patient was urged to severely cut down both alcohol and coffee, and eat regular meals of cooked food. Several weeks later the patient had significantly less gas and had more energy.

Case 6
A patient had explosive diarrhea, swelling of the ankles, colitis, diverticulitis, aversion to cold and heat, and intolerance to fat (her gallbladder had been removed). Her practitioner asked whether to use Mobility 2 or AC-Q. I recommended instead Quiet Digestion and Stomach Tabs in order to remove Dampness and to avoid wasting tonics, herbs which I was afraid she wouldn't be able to absorb.

Case 7
A forty-four year-old client with a biomedical diagnosis of Crohn's disease came in for intractable diarrhea that was only partially alleviated by her medications. The diarrhea caused her considerable worry and fear as she had to be near a bathroom at all times and was always afraid of having an accident; this is common with Crohn's patients. Furthermore, she had extreme fatigue at night. She had been on 80 mg of prednisone for three months within the past year, and was currently taking asulfazine (which was making her sick), and Flagyl. Her tongue was pale, and her pulse slippery. She had a fairly healthy diet and was not taking any dairy products, but was drinking coffee. I explained to her that our allergies are often our addictions, and that she should try to get off coffee and substitute tea. I recommended that she take the Source Qi formula until the diarrhea cleared up, and simultaneously start taking Quiet Digestion after meals, and start taking Six Gentlemen, one tablet TID, and build up to three tablets TID over a two-week period. Within three weeks the diarrhea was not gone. I had her continue with the Quiet Digestion, but substituted Isatis Cooling and Phellostatin for the Source Qi formula and the Six Gentlemen. Although there were no evident Heat signs, there must have been local inflammation. After taking Isatis Cooling and Phellostatin for two weeks her diarrhea and fatigue were improved.

Diabetes

Western Medicine

Differentiation must be made whether patient is insulin or non-insulin dependent.

Astra Essence
Restorative Herbal Formula

Ingredients

English	pinyin
Astragalus root	Huang Qi
Astragalus seed	Sha Yuan Ji Zi
Ligustrum	Nu Zhen Zi
Ho-shou-wu	He Shou Wu
Lycium fruit	Gou Qi Zi
Rehmannia	Shu Di Huang
Eucommia	Du Zhong
Cuscuta	Tu Si Zi
Ginseng	Ren Shen
Tang-kuei	Dang Gui
Cornus	Shan Zhu Yu

(see also: Nine Flavor Tea, Fertile Garden)

TCM

Diabetes almost always involves Yin deficiency. It can be caused by emotional disturbance leading to Liver Qi stagnation, causing Heat. Overeating leads to Damp Heat causing Stomach Fire, which in turn damages the Yin. Over-fatigue or excessive sex causes Kidney Yin and Yang deficiency.

Chinese Herbal Therapy

Insulin dependent diabetes cannot be cured with Chinese herbal therapy; however the symptoms can be alleviated. Non-insulin dependent diabetes can be successfully treated with Chinese herbal medicine.

Good results have been obtained using Astra Essence by itself; it contains several herbs, including Astragalus and Ginseng, which have been shown to reduce serum glucose levels. Additional benefits may be obtained from Nine Flavor Tea, which contains additional Yin tonics. Therefore, these two formulas taken together treat Yin deficiency, Yang deficiency (thus tonifying Yin within Yang), and consolidate the Essence. This combination will treat Heat in the extremities, low back ache, and excessive thirst and urination. A minimum of two tablets of each formula TID must be administered.

If the patient has poor digestion, substitute Fertile Garden for Nine Flavor Tea; Fertile Garden does not contain cooked rehmannia (Shu Di Huang), which can be difficult for American patients to digest.

Case Studies
Case 1: Adult-onset

In one case reported to me by a colleague, a middle-aged woman was able to reduce her glucose levels significantly by taking Astra Essence for about one month at the normal dosage of three tablets TID. Astra Essence contains many herbs such as Rehmannia, Ginseng, Astragalus, and Eucommia which have been shown to reduce glucose levels in experimental research conducted in China.

Case 2: Childhood-onset

A thirty-two year-old man with childhood-onset diabetes, with night sweats, and afternoon facial flushing, fatigue, muscle cramps in the legs, and candidiasis, obtained excellent results for the fatigue and night sweats by taking two tablets of Nine Flavor Tea TID, and two tablets of Astra Essence TID. However, the muscle cramps were not abated.

I suggested trying the AC-Q formula two tablets TID. This patient will have to be monitored to make sure the AC-Q formula is not too warming, and that the Nine Flavor Tea, used for his Yin deficient signs, did no damage to his Stomach and Spleen.

Diarrhea / Food Poisoning

Western Medicine

Loss of fluids from diarrhea can lead to dehydration and loss of minerals. Chronic diarrhea usually indicates an underlying chronic disorder and should be thoroughly diagnosed. Evaluate for food allergies.

TCM

Acute diarrhea is usually due to food stagnation and Dampness. Chronic diarrhea is usually due to Spleen Qi deficiency, or Damp Heat invading the Intestines. Spleen and Kidney Yang deficiency may also be indicated.

Chinese Herbal Therapy

(See also the appendix: Chinese Herbal Treatment of Chronic Digestive Disorders.)

For acute symptoms, Quiet Digestion, formulated with herbs for food stagnation and Dampness, has been specially developed to stop diarrhea and borborygmus. A research formula, Source Qi formula, has been developed to treat severe diarrhea associated with depleted Source Qi, characterized by extreme deficiency of the Spleen and Stomach, anal prolapse, loss of appetite, undigested food in the stool, fluids not being absorbed and "passing straight through," extreme thirst, insufficient fluids, weight loss, wasting of the limbs, fever, and chills. This is found in the later stage of AIDS and other serious disorders.

In chronic diarrhea one must ascertain whether it is due to Spleen Qi deficiency or Damp Heat. The tongue coating with Spleen Qi deficiency is white, but with Damp Heat it will be yellow. Fever or feverish feeling may be present in Damp Heat but not in Qi deficiency. Pulse is slow with Qi deficiency but with Damp Heat it is rapid. Damp Heat is often due to diet rich in heating foods such as fats, sweets, alcohol, and dairy. Spleen Qi deficiency is brought about by excessive eating of cold and raw foods, or by overwork.

Six Gentlemen is useful for Spleen Qi deficient diarrhea, whereas Phellostatin is useful for Spleen Qi deficiency with Damp Heat diarrhea. This syndrome underlies candida infection (see Candidiasis), and includes afternoon feverishness, tiredness, history of eating greasy foods and drinking alcohol. GB-6 is useful when detecting Liver and Gallbladder Heat in the tongue area, with simultaneous Damp Heat.

Traditionally diarrhea in the early morning is called "cock crow" diarrhea and indicates Kidney Yang deficiency. In this case Backbone would be appropriate if there is accompanying weak pulse, loss of appetite, gas, and bloating after meals.

Case Studies

Case 1

A female HIV patient with Cryptosporidium was administered Source Qi and Artestatin by her practitioner. Within six weeks her diarrhea was considerably improved and the Cryptosporidium was eliminated.

Case 2

A thirty-three year-old woman with a high-pressure job came in complaining of constant diarrhea in the morning, with occasional urgent diarrhea during the day. Her pulses were wiry, and her tongue normal-colored. Her medical doctor diagnosed her with Irritable Bowel Syndrome (IBS).

The patient was counseled to eat breakfast, even if it was a few crackers, and to take one tablet of Quiet Digestion every few hours after waking.

After a week, the diarrhea

Quiet Digestion
Shen Chu Gu Ya Herbal Formula

Ingredients

English	*pinyin*
Poria	Fu Ling
Coix	Yi Yi Ren
Shen Chu	Shen Qu
Magnolia	Hou Po
Angelica	Bai Zhi
Pueraria	Ge Gen
Red Atractylodes	Cang Zhu
Saussurea	Mu Xiang
Pogostemon	Huo Xiang
Oryza	Gu Ya
Trichosanthes root	Tian Hua Fen
Chrysanthemum	Ju Hua
Halloysite	Chi Shi Zhi
Citrus	Ju Hong
Mentha	Bo He
Malt	Mai Ya

(see also: Six Gentlemen, Source Qi, Phellostatin, GB-6, Clearing)

---

considerably lessened. She was then told to take two tablets of Quiet Digestion and two tablets of Six Gentlemen TID. After two weeks her diarrhea was improved ninety percent.

Edema

Western Medicine

Edema is fluid that accumulates in the connective tissue. It may be due to a wide variety of causes, and often accompanies serious conditions such as kidney disease, congestive heart failure, and cirrhosis of the liver.

TCM

Edema can be caused by Kidney and Spleen Yang deficiency, and also by exogenous factors which interfere with the Lung's regulation of surface of the body.

Chinese Herbal Therapy

Water's Way addresses Spleen deficiency edema. This formula also successfully treats buildup of fluids due to pathogenic factors. It promotes urination to relieve excess fluids. The basis of this formula is Wu Lin San with the addition of Atractylodes (Bai Zhu) and Stephania (Han Fang Ji), thus increasing the drying and draining effects of the formula.

For Spleen deficiency, this formula may be combined with Six Gentlemen, or with Rehmannia 8 for Kidney Yang deficiency.

If there is lower-body edema, Mobility 2, based on Shu Jing Huo Xue Tang (Clematis and Stephania) can be used by itself, or along with Water's Way. Mobility 2 is usually used for pain associated with arthritis, gout, and sciatica.

Water's Way

Ingredients

English	pinyin
Water Plantain rhizome	Ze Xie
Poria	Fu Ling
Polyporus	Zhu Ling
Stephania	Han Fang Ji
Red Atractylodes	Cang Zhu
White Atractylodes	Bai Zhu
Cinnamon twig	Gui Zhi

(see also: Six Gentlemen, Rehmannia 8, Mobility 2)

Case Study

A 250 pound female patient in her early sixties with arthritis and edema reported that when standing on her feet for long periods, such as when she went shopping, they became extremely painful and swollen. I suggested a combination of Water's Way, one tablet TID, and Mobility 2, three tablets TID. I told her to increase the dosage of Water's Way to three tablets TID when on her feet for long periods. She reported less pain and swelling next time she went shopping.

Endometriosis

Western Medicine

Endometriosis can cause extreme pain in the uterus, lower back, and organs in the pelvic cavity before and during the menses, as well as intermittent pain throughout the menstrual cycle, painful intercourse, excessive bleeding and clots, nausea, vomiting, and constipation during the menses. Endometriosis can also cause infertility.

TCM

Endometriosis can be caused by Heat, Cold, Blood or Qi stagnation.

Chinese Herbal Therapy

With Cold signs, Crampbark Plus is useful for invigorating Blood and alleviating pain. The Unlocking formula is useful for Heat signs. Good results have been obtained using one of the above mentioned formulas with Turtle Shell Tablets, which is based on a research formula used in China. The recommended dosage is two tablets TID or QID. These formulas can be used for alleviating pain and normalizing endometrial tissue. The formulas should be taken for several months, and evaluated regularly, as all three formulas contain dispersing herbs. Tonics such as Astra Essence or Eight Treasures may be used with the formulas if there are signs of tiredness or fatigue.

Turtle Shell Tablets

Ingredients

English	pinyin
Turtle Shell	Bie Jia
Rhubarb	Da Huang
Succinum	Hu Po

(see also: Crampbark Plus, Unlocking)

Fibromyalgia

Western Medicine

Fibromyalgia is chronic pain affecting the ligaments, tendons, and muscles. It occurs mainly in females and may be associated with a pattern of stress (physical or mental), insomnia, trauma (including strenuous exercise), or exposure to dampness or cold. Fibromyalgia may be triggered by a viral infection, and sometimes there is an underlying rheumatic disorder. In men, fibromylagia is more often confined to a local set of muscles, and due to repetitive stress from work-related activity or exercise.

It is important to engage in low- or non-impact aerobic exercises such as walking and swimming. Avoiding repetitive motion is also important, as is stress reduction.

TCM

Fibromyalgia may be due to Qi and Blood stagnation, or an imbalance of Liver and Spleen.

AC-Q Tabs	
Ingredients	
English	*pinyin*
Clematis	Wei Ling Xian
Ginseng	Ren Shen
Siler	Fang Feng
Saussurea	Mu Xiang
Ho-shou-wu	He Shou Wu
Rehmannia	Shu Di Huang
Lindera	Wu Yao
Chiang-huo	Qiang Huo
Tang-kuei	Dang Gui
Gastrodia	Tian Ma
Cinnamon bark	Rou Gui
Aquilaria	Chen Xiang
Frankincense	Ru Xiang
Coptis	Huang Lian
Blue Citrus	Qing Pi
Cloves	Ding Xiang
Gentiana	Qin Jia
Achyranthes	Niu Xio
Loranthus	Sang Ji Sheng
Borneol	Bing Pian
Asarum	Xi Xin

(see also: Clear Heat, Astra Isatis, Ease 2, Ease Plus, Calm Spirit, Schizandra Dreams)

Chinese Herbal Therapy

For fibromyalgia due to virus, Clear Heat has produced excellent results in HIV and CFIDS patients with Heat signs. Astra Isatis should also be used for long range administration for its tonic effects.

AC-Q may be useful is there are signs of Blood stagnation, characterized by sharp stabbing pain, and/or signs of Qi stagnation, characterized by dull achy pain. AC-Q contains tonic herbs and herbs for the above-mentioned patterns.

If stress is a large component, Ease 2 and Ease Plus will address the Liver overacting upon the Spleen/Stomach. Ease 2 is better for stress associated with loose stools and fatigue, whereas Ease Plus is more useful if there is constipation or normal stools. Calm Spirit may be used with Ease 2 and Ease Plus if there is a pattern of insomnia, hot extremities, rapid pulse, or red tongue (see also: Stress and Anxiety). Schizandra Dreams may be used with acute insomnia.

The above-mentioned formulas may be combined.

Case Study

A woman in her late thirties with fibromyalgia was taking several pharmaceutical medications. She had a tremendous number of Heat signs, a full pulse, a yellow coated tongue, and signs of Liver Fire. I recommended three tablets of Coptis Purge Fire every four hours. Within two weeks almost all her symptoms had decreased. Follow-up therapy will probably consist of using a formula such as Astra Isatis, because (acute) symptoms occur because of deficiency.

Gallbladder Stones and Inflammation

Western Medicine

When the gallbladder becomes inflamed, the patient has severe pain in the upper right abdomen. Fried or fatty foods can precipitate an attack. About 10% of acute gall bladder attacks include gangrene and perforation, a potentially fatal medical emergency. Gallstones are usually chronic and are asymptomatic for long periods between attacks of pain.

TCM

Damp Heat in the Liver and Gallbladder. This is a very common syndrome in American women over forty, due to dietary and lifestyle factors. Stones are considered extreme Dampness in Chinese medicine.

Chinese Herbal Therapy

(See also the appendix: Chinese Herbal Treatment of Chronic Digestive Disorders.)

GB-6 has been developed to treat gallbladder stones and gallbladder inflammation. It is based on an empirical formula used in China. Generally the course of treatment is three months. GB-6 may be taken between acute attacks. During acute attacks acupuncture, herbal decoctions, or Western medicine may be indicated. This formula is also useful for women going through rapid weight loss, because they have a propensity for stone build-up.

GB-6

Ingredients

English	pinyin
Ji Nei Jin	Ji Nei Jin
Curcuma	Yu Jin
Corydalis	Yan Hu Suo
Taraxacum	Pu Gong Ying
Melia	Chuan Lian Zi
Salvia	Dan Shen

Case Study

A forty year-old woman approximately twenty pounds overweight complained of nausea and dull aches below the diaphragm several times a day; this was partially relieved by eating. She also had stomach flus every two weeks. Salads, alcohol, and coffee upset her stomach consistently, and she frequently ate fast food and drank diet sodas. She also had PMS and severe menstrual cramps. Her tongue had a greasy coating and her pulse was wiry.

I recommended a medical checkup, and suggested a combination of Woman's Balance and GB-6. Eating greasy and fatty food leads to Damp Heat. Nausea and vomiting are caused by Dampness preventing Stomach Qi from descending and stagnant Liver Qi overacting upon the Stomach. Qi stagnation was evident from the dull aches and PMS. The GB-6 formula was used to remedy Qi and food stagnation, as well as Damp Heat. Woman's Balance was further used for Liver Qi stagnation with Heat. She took two tablets of GB-6 TID, and one tablet of Woman's Balance TID every day. I also recommended that she eliminate diet sodas and fast food, and that she take Quiet Digestion for acute symptoms.

After six weeks she reported considerably less nausea and fewer dull aches despite only a slight reduction in diet sodas and fast food. At this point her tongue was less greasy. She said she would continue to take the herbs.

Headaches

Western Medicine

The most important categories in Western medicine are tension headaches and migraine headaches. A small percentage of headaches are secondary to other illness, sometimes serious; so severe, frequent, or persistent headaches should receive a full medical workup.

TCM Syndromes

May be Wind Heat, Wind Cold, Yang deficiency, Yin deficiency, Internal Wind, Liver Fire rising, Dampness, Blood stasis. Phlegm accumulation, excess Liver Yang, Kidney Yang deficiency, Kidney Yin deficiency.

Chinese Herbal Therapy

It is crucial to differentiate the headache in order to get satisfactory results. If there is a headache due to external pathogens, the onset of the headache is quick and the headache is very painful. Treatment is concerned with expelling the pathogens. If the headache is due to an internal injury there are usually symptoms in the internal organs; then tonic herbs are usually used. If the headache is due to Blood stasis or Phlegm, the excess must be relieved before tonifying.

A Wind Cold headache is characterized by chills and headache. The symptoms are aggravated by wind and cold. There is no thirst or fever, and the tongue coating is thin and white. Recommend three tablets of Head-Q formula with black or green tea every three hours.

Wind Heat headache is characterized by fever, flushed face, thirst, constipation, dark yellow urine, yellow tongue coating, and rapid pulse. Isatis Gold may be applied with chrysanthemum tea every three hours. (see Colds and Flu)

Wind Damp is characterized by heavy-feeling headache, dizziness, poor appetite, and a white greasy tongue coating. Head-Q may be applied with Quiet Digestion.

Excess Liver Yang is caused by emotional disturbances that lead to stagnant Liver Qi which then turns into Fire. Then Yin deficiency of the Liver and Kidney accompanies the excess Liver Yang. Gastrodia Relieve Wind (Gastrodia and Uncaria Formula) can be used along with Coptis Purge Fire if the headache is located in both temples, accompanied by dizziness, irritability, insomnia, bitter taste in the mouth, yellow tongue coating, or red tongue scant coating. Supplement Yin, once Fire is cleared, by using Nine Flavor Tea.

Phlegm accumulation headache is characterized by a heavy-feeling head, nausea, coughing up phlegm, fullness and distension in the chest and abdomen, greasy tongue coat and a slippery pulse. In this case, Gastrodia Relieve Wind taken at three tablets TID, with Lucid Channel at two tablets TID, and Quiet Digestion one tablet before meals (or, with frequent gas, one every two hours) have been very useful.

A headache due to Kidney Yang deficiency is characterized by "empty" feeling headache, dizziness, tinnitus, soreness and weakness of the lower back, coldness. Rehmannia 8 or Backbone formula may be used.

A headache due to Kidney Yin deficiency will have Heat signs and should be treated with Nine Flavor Tea.

A headache due to Qi and Blood deficiency will express itself as chronic headache with fatigue, palpitations, shortness of breath, pale

---

Head-Q
Feverfew with Chinese Aromatics

Ingredients

English	Latin/*pinyin*
Chrysanthemum	Ju Hua
Chiang-huo	Qiang Huo
Ophiopogon	Mai Men Dong
Angelica	Bai Zhi
Ligusticum	Chuan Xiong
Siler	Fang Feng
Scute	Huang Qin
Tang-kuei	Dang Gui
Ginger	Gan Jiang
Asarum	Xi Xin
Raw Rehmannia	Sheng Di Huang
Vitex	Man Jing Zi
Kao-pen	Gao Ben
Licorice	Gan Cao
Feverfew	Tanacetum parthenium

(see also: Isatis Gold, Quiet Digestion, Gastrodia Relieve Wind, Coptis Purge Fire, Nine Flavor Tea, Lucid Channel, Rehmannia 8, Eight Treasures) tongue, weak pulse, and dizziness while standing; use Eight Treasures. Eight Treasures may also be used if these symptoms are seen postmenstrually.

A headache due to Blood stasis is characterized by a dark purple tongue. This usually occurs following a traumatic head injury. Flavonex increases circulation to the head; Resinall K may also be given, in conjunction with medical treatment.

Case Studies

Case 1

A patient came into the clinic with terrible headaches that felt like a tight band was around his head. The headaches were so severe the patient could barely work. He also had persistent postnasal drip. He was told by a neurologist that he had a cholesterol tumor in his head. As an adolescent, he had taken antibiotics for several years to curb acne. We suggested therapies for resolving Dampness and internal Wind. Specifically, Gastrodia Relieve Wind was recommended at three tablets TID, Lucid Channel at two tablets TID, and Quiet Digestion every two hours. Lucid Channel is a very drying formula and it was recommended that the patient take it for three to four weeks. At that point the patient had considerable improvement in the severity of the headaches. The patient was then switched to Quiet Digestion, two tablets TID, and Phellostatin, gradually increasing to three tablets TID between meals over a two week period (i.e. 1 tablet TID the first few days, 2 tablets TID the next few days). After two months patient's headaches were considerably improved, and there was no more postnasal drip. Herbal therapy will continue, using the Flavonex with the Quiet Digestion in order to attempt to resolve the cholesterol growth.

Case 2

Another patient was a hard working "type A" man, who had chronic headaches for years. Although he described the headaches as sinus headaches, they did not get worse upon bending over as is common with sinus headaches, nor did there appear to be any nasal blockage. Nasal dripping only occurred in the fall. This patient often went for four to six days before having a hard, dry bowel movement. He rarely got more than five hours of sleep per night. The tongue was pale with a thin yellow coat. His pulse was weak. At first we used three tablets of Calm Spirit and one tablet of Coptis Purge Fire TID. In my experience, to alleviate the headaches in this type of patient, it is necessary to get the patient to have a normal bowel movement. Calm Spirit was selected as it has a moistening effect on the Intestines, and helps the patient feel more relaxed. The Coptis Purge Fire was suggested as it would further drain Heat.

After one week the patient reported that he began to have more frequent bowel movements. After two to three weeks his headaches were lessened. Follow-up therapy consisted of withdrawing Coptis Purge Fire and substituting Astra Essence to tonify the Kidney. He will take two tablets TID, along with two tablets of Calm Spirit TID.

Hepatitis

Western Medicine

Currently known are Type A, B, C, D, and E hepatitis. The liver may also be damaged by viruses such as herpes simplex or chicken pox virus, or by mononucleosis, particularly when the immune system is compromised. Hepatitis may also be caused by non-viral agents such as chemicals, alcohol, pharmaceutical and recreational drugs.

TCM

In the jaundice stage, characterized by bright yellow skin color, fatigue, restlessness, scanty dark urine, fever, thirst, dry stools, and red tongue with yellow coating, Heat and Dampness must be cleared.

In the chronic stage with loose stools, poor appetite, greasy tongue coat and slow pulse, Qi deficiency, Dampness, and Yang deficiency must be addressed. Other signs may exhibit: Liver Qi stagnation, Damp Heat in the Liver and Gallbladder, and Blood stagnation.

Chinese Herbal Therapy

Because Isatis formulas are widely used in China to treat Hepatitis, Clear Heat, which consists of antiviral herbs, is usually part of the therapy. It can be combined with Coptis Purge Fire, in conjunction with medical treatment for the jaundice stage. The dosage is two tablets of each formula every two to three hours.

In the chronic stage, Ecliptex is usually administered along with other herbs and medical treatment. Ecliptex contains Milk Thistle (Silybum marianum), Eclipta (Han Lian Cao) and other herbs that have been shown to reduce SGPT and SGOT levels on the basis of laboratory experiments conducted in China and Europe. Eclipta is widely used in China and India and thought to be the most powerful liver protectant and regenerative herb available.

With signs of high viral activity, Ecliptex is usually combined with Astra Isatis or Enhance and Clear Heat. Astra Isatis is used when there are signs of Yin and Yang deficiency; Enhance is the formula of choice with if there is Yin, Yang, Qi, and Blood deficiency and Blood stagnation. As mentioned elsewhere, Enhance and Astra Isatis can be switched after several months, as they contain different ingredients, and switching will give the body a break.

Pending grant money, a hundred-patient study has been accepted at a major medical center to study the effects of a combination of Ecliptex, Clear Heat, and Enhance with chronic Hepatitis C. The usual dosage is 20 tablets per day of Enhance, 9 tablets per day of Ecliptex, and 8 tablets of Clear Heat four or five times per day. If Astra Isatis is used instead of Enhance, 12 tablets per day can be used.

Ecliptex
Liver Protection Formula

Ingredients

English	Latin/*pinyin*
Eclipta concentrate	Han Lian Cao
Milk Thistle seed	Silybum marianum
Curcuma	Yu Jin
Salvia	Dan Shen
Lycium Fruit	Gou Qi Zi
Ligustrum	Nu Zhen Zi
Bupleurum	Chai Hu
Schizandra	Wu Wei Zi
Tienchi Ginseng	San Qi
Tang-kuei	Dang Gui
Plantago seed	Che Qian Zi
Licorice	Gan Cao

(see also: Clear Heat, Coptis Purge Fire, Enhance, Astra Isatis)

Case Studies
Case 1

A patient with chronic Hepatitis C was put on a combination of Ecliptex, Enhance, and Clear Heat by her practitioner. The results were so promising that her medical doctors are interested in doing a research project with Chinese herbs and acupuncture. Generally, chronic hepatitis patients take Ecliptex three tablets TID, Enhance four tablets TID, and Clear Heat one to two tablets TID, more if the liver enzymes are rising, or if there are rising Heat signs in terms of TCM.

Case 2

A sixty year-old woman with Hepatitis C had SGOT and SGPT levels twice the normal rate for three months after her diagnosis. Within two months of taking Ecliptex, two tablets TID, both levels dropped to the normal range. She continued to take Ecliptex and her SGOT and SGPT were still within the normal range three months later.

Her liver enzyme readings were as follows:

8/10/92	SGOT	22
	SGPT	16
1/4/93	SGOT	87
	SGPT	82
2/1/93	SGOT	65
	SGPT	95
2/26/93	SGOT	98
	SGPT	148

3/10/93	Started taking Ecliptex
	SGOT 87
	SGPT 118
5/05/93	SGOT 38
	SGPT 36

Herpes (HPV)

Western Medicine

Herpes simplex is a viral infection. After the initial infection the virus becomes dormant in the nerve ganglia, and recurs following minor infections, trauma, stress, and sun exposure. A mild tingling and burning usually precedes genital herpes. This is known as the prodromal stage. Within a few hours blisters develop. Male and female patients may both have a low grade fever and muscular aches. After a few days pus erupts from the blisters and ulcers form.

TCM

Toxic Heat, Heat in the Liver and Gallbladder

Chinese Herbal Therapy

This is an area where merging Chinese and Western Medicine is much stronger than using either alone. Acylovir prevents outbreaks in 91% of patients, but when it is withdrawn, a more serious outbreak may occur. In addition, Acylovir is expensive. We have had extremely encouraging results using the Astra Isatis at the prodromal stage at nine tablets at once, which may need to be repeated. In many cases the outbreak can be prevented. If the outbreak occurs Coptis Purge Fire, based on Long Dan Xie Gan Tang, should be taken, three tablets every two to three hours. Maintenance therapy during the dormant phase is Astra Isatis, three tablets TID, and Power Mushrooms, one tablet TID. With Heat signs use Astra Isatis, three tablets TID, plus Clear Heat, one or two tablets TID. Clear Heat contains antiviral herbs and thus is useful in controlling the active virus. (See also the appendix: Antiviral Properties of Clear Heat.)

Case Studies

Case 1

A male practitioner with genital herpes took nine tablets of Astra Isatis at the prodromal stage of a genital herpes outbreak. This stage is characterized by sensations of itching and feelings of Heat in the outbreak area. The outbreaks usually occur twelve hours to two days later.

The practitioner noticed an abatement of prodromal symptoms a few hours after taking the Astra Isatis, so he took another nine tablets, and the outbreak was completely eliminated.

Since his report I have recommended this protocol often. I usually suggest the genital or oral herpes patient take Astra Isatis, three tablets TID, with either Power Mushrooms with Cold signs or Clear Heat with Heat signs, at one to three tablets TID, for prevention. This tonifies the immune system and attacks the latent virus.

In many cases this seems to reduce the number of outbreaks. In the event patients feel an outbreak coming on, they need to take nine tablets at once. Oftentimes this doesn't need to be repeated. If the outbreak occurs anyway, they should use three tablets of Coptis Purge Fire every two to three hours. This reduces the severity of the outbreaks.

Results have been so positive we are exploring the possibility of a research project in this area. If you are interested in participating as an administrator, please write to me c/o the publisher.

Astra Isatis	
Astragalus & Isatis Extract Formulation	
Ingredients	
English	*pinyin*
Isatis extract	Da Qing Ye and Ban Lan Gen
Astragalus	Huang Qi
Bupleurum	Chai Hu
Laminaria	Kun Bu
Codonopsis	Dang Shen
Epimedium	Yin Yang Huo
Lycium fruit	Gou Qi Zi
Dioscorea	Shan Yao
Broussonetia	Chu Shi Zi
Actractylodes	Bai Zhu
Licorice	Gan Cao

(see also: Coptis Purge Fire, Power Mushrooms, Clear Heat)

We are also using these formulas with herpes zoster, although there have not been as many case studies. Herpes zoster (shingles) patients have responded well to large doses of Clear Heat, three tablets every two hours during the muscle aches associated with the virus. Usually these patients tend to be very deficient, which is why the Astra Isatis is usually recommended along with Clear Heat. The dosage is the same as with herpes simplex in the maintenance stage.

Case 2

One patient, who rarely had herpes simplex outbreaks, was having severe aches in muscles. Medical specialists and doctors at a university hospital told him there was nothing that could be done for his pain other than pain killers. He was put on a combination of Astra Isatis and Clear Heat, two tablets of each QID. In two weeks his muscle aches were substantially reduced and the amount of pain killers he had to consume was reduced by 75%. The patient made even more progress in the following two weeks.

Case 3

A practitioner called to say that a patient with persistent cold sores got relief from Astra Isatis, but they came back as soon as the formula was discontinued. I called and asked how long the patient had been taking Astra Isatis and was told for two weeks.

Analysis: Astra Isatis is very effective at the prodromal stage for cold sores and must be taken at nine tablets at once. If it is taken preventively, it must be taken for several months. The patient appeared deficient so I suggested he take Power Mushrooms in addition to the Astra Isatis. (Use Clear Heat with excess Heat signs). After three months on the full dosage, I suggested trying to reduce the dosage gradually instead of completely eliminating the formula.

Case 4

A thirty-nine year-old man with genital herpes for the last fifteen years who was taking Acyclovir to suppress the outbreaks came in complaining of prodromal symptoms, i.e. sore legs, buttocks, and genital area every day. His practitioner had previously recommended Astra Isatis and it initially worked well, but eventually stopped working, even at three tablets TID. His practitioner had then recommended Bupleurum and Rehmannia Formula but that had stopped working after several weeks. More recently he had taken up to six tablets of Coptis Purge Fire (Gentiana Formula) TID, and after a few weeks that had also ceased being effective.

Unfortunately I have often seen it happen with virally-infected patients that you have to keep rotating formulas as the body becomes "used" to a particular formula. It had been several weeks since he had taken any tonic therapy and I was concerned that his Spleen would be deficient from taking so many cooling herbs. Therefore I recommended a combination of antiviral herbs, with immune tonifying herbs. I suggested two tablets of Clear Heat, two tablets Astra Isatis, and one tablet of Power Mushrooms TID-QID. If he began to feel this protocol losing effectiveness, I suggested he increase the dosage of Clear Heat until he was taking six tablets TID, at which point I suggested another protocol. The second protocol was Isatis Gold and Coptis Purge Fire, starting at two tablets of each TID, with four tablets of Enhance TID. It was my hope that by taking tonic formulas such as Astra Isatis, Power Mushrooms, and Enhance, this patient could get to the point where his immune system was tonified, and begin to see a reduction of prodromal symptoms after a few weeks.

Case 5

A female patient in her forties with a history of cancer who had received a bone marrow transplant two years ago, developed shingles due to her immune-compromised state. Her medical doctor prescribed Acylovir, which dried up the vesicles but seemed to increase the pain. She was very depressed, and wanted to stay in bed and weep all day.

After taking Astra Isatis, two tablets TID, and Clear Heat, four tablets TID, and receiving five acupuncture treatments over two weeks, her energy levels and depression were much better although she continued to need Advil to reduce her pain.

At this point I suggested reducing the Clear Heat, because her tongue was showing more coating and less Heat. I suggested introducing Power Mushrooms, one tablet TID, and increasing the dosage of Astra Isatis to three tablets TID. Follow-up therapy should involve eliminating Clear Heat (which is often effective for reducing pain due to virus), and introducing Marrow Plus to help regenerate bone marrow, and continuing on Astra Isatis and Power Mushrooms. Nine Flavor Tea maybe administered if signs of Heat return, but most of her signs indicated Cold.

Case 6

A colleague saw a patient with cancer that had been in remission who was complaining of superficial headaches and was medically diagnosed with herpes zoster of the eye, for which she was given cortisone. She wanted acupuncture and herbs to avoid a nerve block operation.

The patient was first given homeopathic herpes zoster which didn't help. A few days later she was put on Head-Q and Xanthium Relieve

Surface, three tablets of each formula TID. She was also put on Astra Essence, three tablets BID, since she was Spleen and Kidney deficient. Within two weeks of taking the herbs the patient's husband reported that she needed significantly less pharmaceutical pain relievers.

Analysis: Xanthium Relieve Surface can effectively treat disorders at the surface level. This is why this formula is effective for hayfever, as well as for poison oak and some skin rashes. Head-Q treats upper body tension, and also can be used to treat sinus congestion and itching eyes.

Case 7: *Herpes varicella* paralysis

A woman in her early forties woke up one morning and was paralyzed from the neck down. The medical doctors guessed that she had gotten an infection from the chickenpox virus, which her children had at the time. They said she would never regain any movement.

After a few months of physical therapy she was able to move her upper body, and when she came into my colleague's office her back had spasms, her lower body was atrophied, she felt cold all over, had a bowel movement only once every few days, and had extremely limited range of motion in her hands.

My colleague used ear points, moxibustion, and a combination of AC-Q and Astra Essence, two tablets of each TID. Within a week, she had daily bowel movements, felt warmer, had better energy, and began to get sensations in her legs.

High Blood Pressure

Western Medicine

Hypertension is indicated by repeated blood pressure readings of greater than 150/90 mm Hg. It is estimated that 20% of the adult white male population, and 30% of the black population suffer from hypertension. The usual symptoms are dizziness, vertigo, tinnitus, insomnia, headache, and blurred vision, although these symptoms are not always present. Standard medical therapy involves antihypertensive medication. Although there are many side effects, this medication should only be reduced under medical supervision. Sudden removal of beta-blocker medication may cause heart attacks.

TCM

Internal Wind brought about by rising Heat due to either Liver Fire or deficient Yin/excess Yang. Less common is high blood pressure due to Phlegm and Dampness obstruction or Spleen Qi, and Kidney Yin and Yang deficiency.

Chinese Herbal Therapy

Gastrodia Relieve Wind, also known as Gastrodia and Uncaria Formula, is used to quiet Internal Wind. If there are signs of Liver Fire, such as headache, irritability, facial flushing, bitter taste in the mouth, intense anger, red eyes, constipation with a yellow coated tongue, and a strong rapid pulse, combine Coptis Purge Fire with Gastrodia Relieve Wind, two tablets of each QID.

If there is insomnia, excessive dreaming, dizziness, burning in the soles and palms, night sweats, tinnitus, dry red tongue and rapid pulse, combine Calm Spirit with Gastrodia Relieve Wind, two tablets of each QID. Nine Flavor Tea should be considered as a long-term follow-up for the above mentioned protocols as in the first case the Fire is likely to scorch the Yin, contributing to Yin deficiency, and in any case of Yin deficiency herbs must be used for a long period of time to replenish Yin. If the patient has a weak digestive system, Fertile Garden can be considered, or Nine Flavor Tea can be combined with Quiet Digestion to make the formula more digestible.

It would not be unusual to have high blood pressure with both Liver Fire and Yin deficiency, and therefore a typical protocol may be to use two tablets of Gastrodia Relieve Wind, two tablets of Calm Spirit, and one tablet of Coptis Purge Fire QID. As soon as symptoms begin to clear, withdraw the Coptis Purge Fire and substitute Nine Flavor Tea. After two months or so, use Nine Flavor Tea and Gastrodia Relieve Wind as long-term maintenance.

Signs of Phlegm Damp obstruction include dizziness, nausea, vomiting, and heaviness of the limbs, with chest congestion. Lucid Channel can be combined with Gastrodia Relieve Wind, two tablets of each QID. If there is shortness of breath, fatigue, impotence, frequent urination, Astra 8 may be combined with Astra Essence, two tablets of each TID.

Gastrodia Relieve Wind
Gastrodia and Uncaria Formula

Ingredients

English	pinyin
Gastrodia	Tian Ma
Uncaria	Gou Teng
Abalone shell	Shi Jue Ming
Gardenia	Zhi Zi
Scute	Huang Qin
Leonuris	Yi Mu Cao
Cyathula	Chuan Niu Xi
Eucommia	Du Zhong
Loranthus	Sang Ji Sheng
Polygonum stem	Ye Jiao Teng
Fu-shen	Fu Shen

(see also: Calm Spirit, Nine Flavor Tea, Coptis Purge Fire, Lucid Channel, Astra 8, Astra Essence)

Notes

Obesity is a major factor in hypertension, as is caffeine consumption, smoking, alcohol, lack of exercise, stress, and chronic exposure to lead. These factors must be addressed. A TCM diet low in sodium is also recommended. Biofeedback and acupuncture are very effective. Medical monitoring is necessary.

Case Studies
Case 1

A patient in his early sixties, in good health except for high cholesterol and moderate high blood pressure, was given a combination of Flavonex and Astra Garlic, two tablets of each TID, by his practitioner, along with the suggestion that he adopt a low-fat diet. After six weeks his high blood pressure had dropped ten points, and his cholesterol was down 5%.

Case 2

A man in his late forties with high blood pressure, dizziness, headache and irritability with no pronounced Heat signs was put on Gastrodia Relieve Wind by his practitioner. After four weeks the patient was very happy with the symptomatic results he was getting from the herbs.

Case 3

A man in his late fifties wanted help reducing his high blood pressure. The patient was experiencing headache, dizziness, and sweating. He was put on Gastrodia Relieve Wind, three tablets TID, and within three weeks was reporting considerably less headaches and dizziness. I had pointed out that the sweating could be controlled with other herbs, but he was reluctant to take any more tablets. He also reported that he was having insomnia and wanted to know if the Gastrodia Relieve Wind contained stimulants. I reported that it didn't, but there were formulas we could use for insomnia such as Schizandra Dreams. It was not clear whether or not the formula actually caused a permanent decrease in his blood pressure or if it only decreased the side effects.

High Cholesterol

Western Medicine

High serum cholesterol is implicated in cerebrovascular and cardiac insufficiency. A high cholesterol diet is also implicated in gallstones, high blood pressure and even in cancer. Western medicine stresses the need for a TCM diet with special attention to staying away from salt. Dietary fiber is very important in reducing cholesterol. A high-fiber diet and anti-cholesterol drugs are the most common forms of treatment.

TCM

Excess meat and fats were seen as a problem by the ancients. Cholesterol can be characterized by Dampness and Blood stagnation.

Astra Garlic

Ingredients

English	pinyin
Odorless Garlic	Da Suan
Astragalus	Huang Qi
Ho-shou-wu (Fo-ti)	He Shou Wu
Ganoderma (Rei-Shi)	Ling Zhi
Crataegus	Shan Zha
Tang-kuei	Dang Gui
Salvia	Dan Shen
White Atractylodes	Bai Zhu

Chinese Herbal Therapy

Garlic, used both in Western and Chinese medicine, has been found to be an excellent therapy for high cholesterol levels; however concern may be raised with certain cardiovascular patients since whole cloves of garlic each day may be excessively warming.

Crataegus (Shan Zha) is traditionally used to counter the effects of meat eating. Ho shou wu has been found to reduce cholesterol, as has ganoderma. Other herbs with circulatory effects include Astragalus, Salvia, Tang-kuei, and White Atractylodes. These herbs are found in Astra Garlic, which contains specially processed, concentrated, odorless garlic.

Notes

Follow TCM diet, emphasizing high fiber. Oat bran and brown rice bran are the best foods for lowering cholesterol. Meat and dairy products, alcohol, and caffeine are major contributing factors to high cholesterol. Steroids, oral contraceptives, diuretics, etc, also cause high cholesterol. Extra virgin cold pressed olive oil is said to reduce cholesterol.

Case Study

A middle-aged man in good health, with some fatigue and high cholesterol levels came in. His pulse was slightly slow, and his tongue slightly pale. He was put on Astra Garlic and advised to start a low-fat, high-fiber diet. After three weeks his cholesterol was significantly lowered.

HIV

Western Medicine

Thousands of individuals with HIV self-medicate with Chinese herbs, Western herbs, and supplements in order to keep themselves healthy. Medical doctors who see significant numbers of HIV-infected patients will encourage or accept alternatives to the standard medical treatment, as they help achieve better sleep, decrease fatigue, and reduce opportunistic infections. Approaches such as acupuncture and herbs should be used in conjunction with Western medical diagnosis, and approved and experimental drugs.

TCM

Qi deficiency, Yin deficiency, digestive complaints, Yang deficiency, Blood deficiency, Blood stagnation, Toxic Heat.

Chinese Herbal Therapy

(See also the appendix: Integrating Chinese Herbs and Western Medicine in the Treatment of HIV.)

In the San Francisco Bay area, Chinese herbs are used by a large percentage of the HIV-infected population. A double-blind study conducted at San Francisco General Hospital compared a combination of two Chinese herbal formulas, Enhance and Clear Heat, with a placebo. Preliminary results indicate that life-satisfaction improved significantly in the Chinese medicine group as compared to the placebo group. Improvement was also observed in fatigue, gastrointestinal symptoms, and neurological symptoms in the herb group vs. the placebo group. There were some symptoms that did not show a difference between the two groups, and dermatological symptoms improved in the placebo group.

Enhance and Clear Heat were developed out of the experience at Quan Yin Clinic in San Francisco, where thousands of HIV-infected patients have been treated with acupuncture and Chinese herbs. Enhance contains Qi, Yin, Yang, and Blood tonics, Blood-activating herbs, and anti-Toxin herbs. Enhance is the base formula, and then specific formulas are added for each patient's symptoms. The typical dosage of Enhance is five tablets QID. Adjuncts are usually taken three tablets TID.

The most frequently used adjunct formula is Clear Heat, which consists largely of anti-Toxin herbs. Anti-Toxin herbs have anti-viral effects as demonstrated in clinical studies conducted in China. Clear Heat is combined with Enhance when patients have a high level of viral activity, or feelings of feverishness or excess Heat.

Marrow Plus is used with Enhance for restoring bone marrow that has been suppressed by AZT or other chemotherapeutic agents. It contains herbs that are considered Blood-activating and Blood-tonifying in terms of TCM.

Quiet Digestion is used by individuals who have digestive difficulties, or problems digesting the herbs. Xanthium Relieve Surface is indicated for patients with sinus allergies or infections. Artestatin has been used with the Source Qi formula for individuals infected by cryptosporidium with chronic watery diarrhea.

Enhance
Quan Yin Herbal Formula

Ingredients

English	pinyin
Ganoderma	Ling Zhi
Isatis extract	Ban Lan Gen and Da Qing Ye
Millettia extract	Ji Xue Teng
Astragalus	Huang Qi
Tremella	Bai Mu Er
Andrographis	Chuan Xin Lian
Lonicera	Jin Yin Hua
Aquilaria	Chen Xiang
Epimedium	Yin Yang Huo
Oldenlandia	Bai Hua She She Cao
Cistanche	Rou Cong Rong
Lycium fruit	Gou Ji Zi
Laminaria	Kun Bu
Tang-kuei	Dang Gui
Hu-chang	Hu Chang
American Ginseng	Xi Yang Shen
Schizandra	Wu Wei Zi
Ligustrum	Nu Zhen Zi
Atractylodes	Bai Zhu
Rehmannia	Shu Di Huang
Salvia	Dan Shen
Curcuma	Yu Jin
Viola	Zi Hua Di Ding
Citrus	Chen Pi
Peony	Bai Shao
Ho-shou-wu	He Shou Wu
Eucommia	Du Zhong
Cardamom	Sha Ren
Licorice	Gan Cao

(see also: Marrow Plus, Clear Heat, Quiet Digestion, Nine Flavor Tea, Source Qi, Celosia 10, Eupolyphaga Tablets)

There have also been reports that Bioradiance is useful for intractable diarrhea in HIV patients. Clear Air is useful to ventilate the Lung, and has been used successfully as an adjunct to antibiotics with pneumonia patients.

Celosia 10 has been used with some success in the early stages of CMV retinitis, at the dosage of five tablets TID. There has also been some success using Colostroplex with CMV-related conditions. Tremella and American Ginseng can be used to treat night sweating.

Those who have had considerable experience in treating HIV-infected patients have found that Chinese herbs do not increase T-4 counts, and may not have a significant effect on other laboratory parameters, although they do improve the quality of life for most people taking well-prescribed formulas.

Notes

It is important to always attack the virus using Clear Heat herbs, regardless of the signs and symptoms according to TCM. This is why Enhance contains antiviral herbs. If Yin deficiency predominates, use a Yin tonic formula such as Nine Flavor Tea.

Case Studies

Case 1

A male HIV-infected patient in his early thirties with extreme fatigue and night sweats started to take Enhance, five tablets TID. Within two weeks, he reported having much more energy. After one month his night sweats were gone. After six months, he reported that he was more energetic than his friends who were not HIV-infected. He attributed this to taking Enhance.

Analysis: Under normal circumstances I would have recommended that he switch to Astra Isatis for one month; he was reluctant to do so. I suggested that he not over-exert himself, despite feeling so well, and maintain healthy lifestyle habits.

Case 2

An otherwise healthy HIV patient had been admitted to the hospital for pneumonia. After several days of intravenous antibiotics, he was released from the hospital and told to check in with the nurse the following day. He went to the Quan Yin clinic and was advised to take Clear Air, three tablets every few hours. When he returned to the hospital, the nurse asked how his lungs had cleared up so much in the past twenty-four hours. He told the nurse he had been taking Chinese herbs. "Nothing works that fast," she replied.

Analysis: Clear Air has powerful expectorants and is a modification of the traditional formula Ding Chuan Tang. It is usually used when there are Heat signs (colored phlegm). This formula has been very successful not only with HIV patients, but with asthmatics and individuals who get frequent attacks of bronchitis.

Case 3

An HIV-infected patient who had T-4's in the 300-400 range started to take Enhance and had a doubling of his T-4's within one month. Patient and practitioner were both very happy.

Three months later when the patient was retested, his T-4's were back in the 300-400 range. Both patient and practitioner were discouraged. The patient's medical doctor urged him to take AZT.

Analysis: Chinese herbs do not lead to a sustained increase in T cells, although, according to Misha Cohen, OMD, LAc, those who take Chinese herbal protocols for extended time periods usually do not decline as fast as those who don't take Chinese herbs. This conclusion is based on clinical and research experience at Quan Yin Clinic. In the particular case mentioned above, I suggested that the practitioner give Marrow Plus if the patient was to go on AZT. I told her of two cases I was familiar with in which AIDS patients taking Chinese herbs with a T-4 count of zero were able to survive outside of the hospital. One of these patients was able to work every day.

What we hope to do using Chinese herbal therapy is to improve the quality of life, rather than improve particular lab results. The case above is sad, because perhaps the patient developed unreasonable expectations of the formula.

I have heard frustration on the part of some practitioners who treat AIDS patients; many patients who come in fatigued and sick get good results with acupuncture, herbs and lifestyle modifications, but then once they are better they stop coming in for treatment, abandon lifestyle modifications, and then return after several months in worse shape than on their initial visit.

I applaud the efforts of those practitioners around the country who are helping to provide ongoing low-cost care to the HIV-infected population.

Case 4

A male HIV patient with a T-4 count below 100, on AZT, complained of severe neuropathy. The pain was so bad he could not sleep for longer than fifteen minutes without waking up.

The primary treatment for this is acupuncture, massage, and moxibustion (if there are no Heat signs). I suggested that the practitioner use Clear Heat along with the above mentioned therapies, since I believed it was the virus lodged in the muscle sheath that was causing the pain, and waking up so frequently is also a sign of extreme Heat. The patient took three tablets Clear Heat TID and also added Enhance to his protocol slowly. Within a day after taking Clear Heat and acupuncture, he reported his pain was significantly reduced.

Case 5

A thirty-five year-old male HIV patient who had been taking Enhance and Clear Heat for six months had been recently on Septra for three months for a bad case of bronchitis. He was also taking prednisone and reported headaches that started behind the eye and spread to the temples, suggesting Heat in the Stomach, Liver, and Gallbladder. I suggested that the patient temporarily discontinue Enhance, and take Gastrodia Relieve Wind and Coptis Purge Fire instead. It was my hypothesis that Wind was invading due to Yin deficiency and fire. The T-4 count was low, suggesting high levels of viral activity.

Prednisone creates Heat, and Septra creates Dampness; these conditions will need to be addressed if the above protocol is not successful.

Impotence

Western Medicine

Peripheral vascular disease, diabetes, alcohol, cigarettes, and psychological factors may all contribute to impotence. Use of certain western drugs, including high blood pressure medications, may also cause impotence.

TCM

Impotence is usually due to Kidney Yang deficiency.

Chinese Herbal Therapy

If there is definite Kidney Yang deficiency with no Heat signs, Backbone is an excellent formula. If the patient has Yin and Yang deficiency, Astra Essence is an excellent choice, because it offers a more balanced therapy. Flavonex, which contains Ginkgo biloba extract, may be used if there is not a clear-cut case of Kidney Yang deficiency, because this herb has been shown effective for men who cannot achieve an erection due to poor circulation.

Patients usually need to take an herbal formula at the full dose for three to

---

Backbone
Bu Shen Huo Xie

Ingredients

English	pinyin
Eucommia	Du Zhong
Psoralea	Bu Gu Zhi
Cibotium	Gou Ji
Cuscuta	Tu Si Zi
Cistanche	Rou Cong Rong
Rehmannia	Shu Di Huang
GuiBan	Gui Ban
Cyathulae	Chuan Niu Xi
Acanthopanacis	Wu Jia Pi
Tang-kuei tails	Dang Gui Wei
Dipsaci	Xu Duan
Carthamis	Hong Hua
Myrrh	Mo Yao
Cornus	Wu Zhu Yu

(see also: Astra Essence, Essence Chamber, Flavonex)

six weeks in order to notice any results.

Case Study

A man in his late fifties complaining of frequent urination and impotence took Astra Essence, three tablets TID. After three weeks he remarked that his potency had returned. After taking Essence Chamber for prostatic hypertrophy, some patients notice this formula also increases their sex drive.

Infertility

Western Medicine

As many as 15% of couples experience the inability to conceive. Male reproductive disorders account for 40% of the cases. Female problems that cause infertility include failure to ovulate (30%), tubal disease or endometriosis (50%), cervical pathology (10%), and unknown causes (10%). Conventional treatment includes drug therapy to induce ovulation, surgical correction of tubal obstruction or adhesions, and *in vitro* fertilization and embryo transfer (effective about a third of the time).

TCM

When not due to anatomical obstruction, female infertility may involve Kidney Yin deficiency, Kidney Yang deficiency, Liver Qi stagnation and other imbalances. The best treatment approach involves monitoring the specific phase in the menstrual cycle, and matching the corresponding TCM signs with a specific formula or formulas.

Chinese Herbal Therapy

If there is Dampness and Phlegm, these should be cleared before any tonification is started. This pattern will be characterized by obesity, delayed menstruation, excessive and sticky leukorrhea, fullness in the chest, dizziness, nausea, white and greasy tongue coating, with a slippery pulse. Lucid Channel is an excellent formula to start with. Typically, once the above pattern has cleared, another one will present. If there is also food stagnation (which is common in obesity), combine Lucid Channel with Quiet Digestion.

For American women in their late thirties or older, Kidney and Liver Yin deficiency may be the predominant pattern. Fertile Garden was developed to address the problems of career women who have led stress-filled lives and want to become pregnant. Since stress creates Liver Qi stagnation, and since Liver Qi stagnation leads to Heat, and Heat exhausts Yin and Blood, the patient may have early and scant periods, dry skin and hair, depression, emotional sensitivity, insomnia, and fatigue.

There may be signs of Liver Qi stagnation either in the premenstrual phase only or as a constitutional imbalance. It is characterized by irritability, anger, and breast fullness, with abdominal pain before menstruation; in this case Woman's Balance can be administered throughout the month or only during the premenstrual period. If a woman cannot maintain a post-ovulatory or luteal phase basal body temperature during the premenstrual phase, this is usually due to Qi deficiency, in which case Arouse Vigor can be administered, or Two Immortals if there is Yang deficiency with deficiency Heat. If there are menstrual cramps Crampbark Plus may be administered.

If the pattern is one of Kidney Yang and Blood deficiency, characterized by delayed menstruation, scant and pale menstrual blood, fatigue, feeling of coldness, and tiredness in the limbs, with pale tongue and slow pulse, Dr. Fung's Fertility Formula will be more effective as this contains several traditional fertility herbs and has proven to be effective over a long period of time.

It is important, as always with Chinese herbs, to treat what you see. It would be possible to use a combination of these formulas simultaneously.

Fertile Garden

Modified One Stack
Fertility Promoting Tablets

Ingredients

English	Latin/*pinyin*
Loranthus	Sang Ji Sheng
Ligustrum	Nu Zhen Zi
Glehnia	Sha Shen
Cuscuta	Tu Si Zi
Pseudostellaria	Tai Zi Shen
Shatavari	Tian Men Dong
Tang-kuei	Dang Gui
White Peony	Bai Shao
Lycium fruit	Gou Ji Zi
Poria	Fu Ling
Ashwagandha	Withaniae somniferae
Melia	Chuan Lian Zi
Baked Licorice	Zhi Gan Cao
Placenta	Zi He Che

(see also: Woman's Balance, Two Immortals, Arouse Vigor, Crampbark Plus, Dr. Fung's Fertility Formula)

Case Study

One of my more complicated consultations was with a TCM practitioner whose patient was undergoing *in vitro* fertilization. The patient was taking a very strong Western drug to stop menstruation so that at the right time another strong Western drug could be given to start menstruation. The practitioner wanted to know what herbs would help this patient, who had a weak constitution.

I asked about her signs and symptoms according to TCM, and the practitioner mentioned Liver Qi stagnation. I suggested Ecliptex, since many Western drugs will cause Liver Qi stagnation. Ecliptex is also the best herbal formula I know of to take as a preventive along with Western drugs that are toxic to the Liver.

Injury

Western Medicine

Western medicine excels at repair of gross injury to the tissues and organs, but has little to offer for less serious injuries such as bruises, internal muscle and connective tissue tears, and swelling due to trauma.

TCM

In the initial stage, 24-36 hours after an injury, there may be Heat (inflammation). Injuries involve Blood stagnation, and in the later stages there can also be Qi stagnation as well as Yin and Yang deficiency.

Chinese Herbal Therapy

Resinall K, based on Qi Li San (without Cinnabar, a toxic mercury compound), relieves pain and activates Blood, and is used for injury treatment. It comes in liquid extract form which is taken under the tongue for fast absorption. Resinall K works well in conjunction with Flavonex, a formula which activates Blood. Flavonex has bioflavonoid-containing herbs which have natural anti-inflammatory properties.

Since there is often swelling at the very first stages of an injury, Yin Chao Jin can be used in addition to these other formulas, if it is within the first three days of the injury. This formula will help reduce swelling. Yin Chao Jin and the other formulas are taken at least three tablets every three to four hours. In addition to Resinall K, AC-Q can be used if there is a lower body injury. If there is an upper body injury use the SPZM formula with Resinall K. SPZM is particularly good with injuries such as whiplash, and can be used for carpal tunnel syndrome as well.

Ease 2 can be used for Liver Qi stagnation, which often occurs during injury.

For long-term treatment of an injury, Flavonex is used with AC-Q, which contains tonic herbs and ingredients for opening the Channels and relieving pain. The circulation of Blood and Qi is promoted to relax muscles and sinews, expelling Wind and Cold, stopping spasm and reducing pain. As a final note to injury treatment, if you are not getting adequate results, you may try AC-Q earlier. Backbone is specifically used for bone weakness. This formula contains bone-knitting herbs. As it contains Kidney Yang tonics it should be modified with Nine Flavor Tea or Temper Fire with those who have any Heat signs.

Case Studies

Case 1

A thirty year-old man fell off his bike and had multiple abrasions, although no broken bones. In addition he was "shaken up." Resinall K was administered immediately, one full dropper under the tongue. He was told to take Resinall K every two hours. He was also given Ease 2, since most of the pain was in the upper body (he had flown over the handlebars). Ease 2 contains herbs such as Pueraria (Ge Gen), which releases the muscles, Bupleurum (Chai Hu), and Cinnamon Twig (Gui Ghi) which releases the exterior. Ease 2 was taken three tablets TID. This formula also has a stress-relieving effect.

After a few days Resinall K had to be withdrawn due to an alcohol sensitivity. He had a history of candidiasis, and Flavonex was substituted. He reported significant symptomatic relief from Resinall K.

Resinall K
Historical Basis Qi Li San
Ingredients

English	Latin/*pinyin*
Dragon's Blood	Xue Jie
Catechu	Er Cha
Corydalis	Yan Hu Suo
Kava	Piper methysticum
Carthamus (Safflower flower)	Hong Hua
Myrrh	Mo Yao
Frankincense	Ru Xiang
Borneol	Bing Pian
Alcohol	

(see also: Flavonex, AC-Q, Yin Chao Jin, Backbone)

Case 2

A former martial-artist in her forties started to take up long distance running and developed severe back problems that were only partially alleviated by massage and chiropractic. I recommended Ease 2, and a week later the patient reported significant relief.

After a few weeks I switched to Ecliptex, because the patient reported that she also had chronic headaches that were only alleviated by an expensive patent medicine from Chinatown containing caffeine, phenobarbital, other chemicals which were not listed on the label but were found on the packaging insert. I suggested using Ecliptex as a constitutional remedy because the patient was Blood deficient, Yin deficient, and had Blood stagnation. I suggested she stop taking the Chinese patent remedy; the pharmaceuticals in patent medicines are of unknown dosage, quality, and amounts. At least with Western pharmaceuticals you know what you are getting. After two months the patient reported fewer headaches, more mental clarity, and significantly less back pain.

Analysis: Ease 2 is very effective for muscle aches that are stress-induced, with Liver Qi stagnation. It is an herbal concentrate for fast relief. Ecliptex was recommended as a follow-up because the patient had dry skin, red tongue in the Liver and Gallbladder areas, pale tongue in other areas, and a pattern of Liver Qi stagnation (unexpressed anger, rigid personality). Finally, due to her fifteen years of martial arts there had to be some Blood stagnation. I initially suggested Ease 2 because she was also having a problem with loose stools, which also cleared up.

Irritable Bowel Syndrome

Western Medicine
Irritable bowel syndrome (IBS), also known as spastic colon, is a condition where the colon (large intestine) does not work correctly. IBS is characterized by abdominal pain with distension and alternating constipation and diarrhea, anxiety, and depression. IBS is not associated with changes to the intestine or inflammation.

TCM
Liver invading the Spleen/Stomach with food stagnation.

Chinese Herbal Therapy
Stomach Tabs, based on Ping Wei San, is modified with Bpluerum since many individuals with this disorder tend to repress their emotions. It is also recommended that patients consume at least three cups of peppermint tea per day.

Case Study
A forty-five year-old woman with history of physical abuse was seen by a colleague and com-

Ease Plus
Bupleurum Plus Combination

Ingredients

English	pinyin
Oystershell calcium	Mu Li and Long Gu
Bupleurum	Chai Hu
Ginseng	Ren Shen
Ginger	Gan Jiang
Pinellia	Ban Xia
Scute	Huang Qin
Cinnamon	Gui Zhi
Rhubarb	Da Huang
Saussurea	Mu Xiang

(see also: Quiet Digestion, Isatis Cooling)

plained of frequent intestinal cramping. She also reported a tight neck, constipation, cold hands and feet and other signs of Liver Qi stagnation. Due to the intestinal cramping, her medical doctor had prescribed frequent rounds of antibiotics, which helped. However, the pain always returned after the course of antibiotics ended. My colleague recommended Isatis Cooling, three tablets TID, which produced a marked reduction in cramping within a few days.

Since the shoulder and neck tension and constipation remained, I suggested using two tablets of Ease Plus and two tablets of Calm Spirit, each TID. The woman was under tremendous stress from an abusive relationship, and this combination of formulas works extremely well with stress related shoulder and neck tension. It also contains ingredients that help move the bowels and smooth Liver Qi. Isatis Cooling was recommended to be used only when she had intestinal complaints.

Kidney Stones

Western Medicine

Ordinarily urine prevents stones from forming. Many of the symptoms of Kidney stones, including severe pain, nausea and vomiting, burning urination, blood in the urine, inability to urinate, cloudy urination, and frequent urination may be associated with other kidney and urinary tract disorders; Western medical diagnosis is therefore very important.

TCM

Symptoms may be due to Qi stagnation, characterized by distending pain that starts in the right upper abdomen, and abdominal distension with no signs of Heat or fever. Damp Heat herbs address continuous radiating or distending pain, with symptoms of Heat. Techniques are also used in Chinese clinics which combine Chinese herbs and Western medicine in order to get stones to pass.

Chinese Herbal Therapy

Treatment in the West usually involves tableted formulas because the treatment period is several months. Formulas usually address several imbalances. Jin Qian Cao Stone Formula will be the subject of a research project at a major medical center in San Francisco.

Jin Qian Cao Stone Formula has specific herbs that are traditionally used to dissolve stones, including Lycimachia (Jin Qian Cao) and Lygoidium (Hai Jin Sha), with herbs to promote urination and Blood circulation. This formula is recommended when the patient has at least four months to wait before surgery is necessary. It is important to realize that, even after surgery, the stones continue to form; therefore this formula might also be used as a preventive after surgery.

Although we know the herbs work, we do not know if they dissolve the stones, or if they help the stones to pass.

Case Studies

Case 1

A fifty year-old man with a 3 cm kidney stone came for treatment. He had an acute kidney infection for a year and a half, a low grade kidney infection for five years, and a history of sexually-transmitted disease (STD). There was a conflict between his general medical doctor and his urologist. The urologist wanted to operate, but the G.P., who was afraid of complications, wanted him to wait. Ultrasound had been tried and had not been successful, and he had been on and off antibiotics for long periods of time for the kidney infection. Sodium bicarbonate had also been used to try shrinking the stone; however, it was not successful.

I recommended a combination of Unlocking and Akebia Moist Heat, two tablets of each QID; this combination of formulas is specific for Damp Heat in the Lower Burner.

Patrinia (Bai Jiang Cao), an ingredient in Unlocking, is specifically used for Lower Burner Heat particularly due to STD. Akebia Moist Heat is excellent for urinary inflammation and discomfort. I used both formulas to get a broad spectrum action. I also suggested he begin Jin Qian Cao Stone Formula as soon as the kidney infection cleared up.

Chronic Dampness is difficult to get rid of. If the kidneys are not working well, it is likely the Spleen and Kidney, in TCM terms, are also not working well. Therefore, this patient had stones and frequent kidney infections. Antibiotics may resolve the infection, but they create more Dampness. This patient will also require long-term Spleen and Kidney tonification.

Jin Qian Cao Stone Formula

Ingredients

English	*pinyin*
Lycimachia	Jin Qian Cao
Lygoidum	Hai Jin Sha
Bupleurum	Chai Hu
Plantago	Che Qian Zi
Polygonum	Bian Xu
Dianthus	Qu Mai
Red Peony	Chi Shao
Gardenia	Zhi Zi
Capillaris	Yin Chen
Chih-shih	Zhi Shi
Tienchi	San Qi
Licorice	Gan Cao

(see also: Unlocking, Akebia Moist Heat)

Case 2

A colleague was treating a forty-six year-old man who was passing kidney stones and was in tremendous pain. He had been prescribed Demerol by his medical doctor. The patient had bloody urine. Acupuncture on bladder points helped with the pain.

I suggested using a combination of Unlocking and Akebia Moist Heat, two tablets of each QID. This combination was used to reduce Damp Heat, Qi stagnation, and Blood stagnation. Although I didn't have enough information to do a complete TCM work-up, blood in the urine is indicative of Heat, and kidney stones are usually a result of Damp Heat. This combination of formulas was directed at the Lower Burner.

Leukorrhea

Western Medicine

Leukorrhea refers to vaginal discharge.

TCM

Leukorrhea is usually categorized into yellow or colored discharge, indicating Heat, or clear or white discharge indicating Cold.

Six Gentlemen
Modified Liu Jun Zi Formula

Ingredients

English	pinyin
Codonopsis	Dang Shen
Atractylodes	Bai Zhu
Poria	Fu Ling
Baked Licorice	Zhi Gan Cao
Citrus	Chen Pi
Pinellia	Ban Xia
Saussurea	Mu Xiang
Cardamon	Sha Ren

(see also: Isatis Cooling, Phellostatin)

Chinese Herbal Therapy

Isatis Cooling is indicated for Hot leukorrhea, whereas Cold leukorrhea is countered by combining Six Gentlemen with Phellostatin. Vagistatin may also be used externally (as a vaginal insert) for Hot leukorrhea.

Case Study

A woman in her early forties, with a demanding job and busy social schedule, complained of fatigue and clear leukorrhea. Her pulse was wiry and her tongue was pale. I suggested Astra Essence and Phellostatin, two tablets of each formula TID. After four weeeks she reported that the leukorrhea was gone and that the fatigue was considerably lessened.

Lumbago (Lower Back Pain)

Western Medicine

Dull lower back pain may be caused by rheumatoid arthritis, muscle strain, trauma, nephritis, and other causes.

TCM

Usually caused by Blood stasis, Cold, and Kidney deficiency.

Chinese Herbal Therapy

For low back pain, weakness in the back and knees, cold limbs, fatigue, pale face and tongue, and slow pulse use Backbone formula, which is based on several traditional formulas.

Astra Essence is more suitable for those who have mixed Cold and Heat signs. Astra Essence contains Lycium (Gou Qi Zi), Cuscuta (Tu Si Zi), and Eucommia (Du Zhong), which are very useful in treating lower back weakness.

For pain that worsens in damp weather, AC-Q is more suitable than the above-mentioned formulas. It can be used for mus-

Backbone Bu Shen Huo Xie	
Ingredients	
English	*pinyin*
Eucommia	Du Zhong
Psoralea	Bu Gu Zhi
Cibotium	Gou Ji
Cuscuta	Tu Si Zi
Cistanche	Rou Cong Rong
Rehmannia	Shou Di Huang
GuiBan	Gui Ban
Cyathulae	Chuan Niu Xi
Acanthopanacis	Wu Jia Pi
Tang-kuei tails	Dang Gui Wei
Dipsaci	Xu Duan
Carthamis	Hong Hua
Myrrh	Mo Yao
Cornus	Wu Zhu Yu
(see also: Astra Essence, Mobility 2)	

cle aches, joint pain, radiating pain in the leg, numbness, pain in the trunk and extremities (see Arthritis).

Case Study

A male client in his mid thirties was mugged and beaten, and received numerous blows to his lower and mid back. His tongue was pale and his pulse weak. He suffered from both dull aches and sharp, stabbing pain. Backbone was recommended, three tablets TID. Within a few days after taking the formula the client reported decreased aches and pains.

Lupus

Western Medicine

Systemic lupus is an autoimmune disease that produces inflammation to the blood vessels and joints. Kidney failure is common in those with systemic lupus. Discoid lupus is a skin disease that causes disfiguration. Certain drugs may cause lupus. Chemicals, pollutants, stress, fatigue, and viral infections that haven't been identified, can also cause lupus.

Anti-inflammatory drugs, corticosteroids, radiation,and even anti-malarial drugs are used in the treatment of lupus. For more information on conventional treatments, call the Lupus Foundation at 1-800-558-0121.

TCM

Heat, Blood stasis, deficient Yin, and sometimes deficient Qi and Yang.

Chinese Herbal Therapy

Lithospermum 15 is a specific formula designed for Lupus; it

Coptis Purge Fire
Ingredients

English	pinyin
Coptis	Huang Lian
Lophatherum	Dan Zhu Ye
Bupleurum	Chai Hu
Rehmannia	Sheng Di Huang
Tang-kuei	Dang Gui
Peony	Bai Shao
Anemarrhena	Zhi Mu
Akebia	Mu Tong
Sophora	Ku Shen
Scute	Huang Qin
Phellodendron	Huang Bai
Gentiana	Long Dan Cao
Forsythia	Lian Qiao
Gardenia	Zhi Zi
Licorice	Gan Cao

(see also: Clear Heat, Ecliptex, Nine Flavor Tea, Lithospermum 15)

clears Toxin, vitalizes Blood, and includes tonic herbs. If there is a sudden onset, high fever, flushed face, red-colored skin rash, irritability, thirst, constipation, scanty and dark urine, arthralgia, and rapid pulse, Coptis Purge Fire may be used, three or more tablets every three hours. Also add one or two tablets of Clear Heat. Clear Heat contains Isatis extract, which is useful to clear Heat Toxin in the Blood.

Ecliptex, which activates Blood and tonifies Liver Yin, combined with Nine Flavor Tea, two tablets of each formula TID, with Clear Heat one or two tablets TID, may be the basis of a good long-term treatment.

Case Study

A forty-four year-old female patient who had only two of the criteria for lupus, including a positive lupus antibody test and aches and pains in the knees and lower back, had been put on a prescription analgesic. However, this drug lowered her kidney function and she sought out acupuncture.

Her tongue was pale, with a white coat, her pulse was slippery and slow. She had fatigue; while standing up she felt weak and had spots before her eyes.

I recommended a combination of Backbone to treat Kidney and Spleen Yang deficiency, and Eight Treasures, to treat Blood and Qi deficiency (i.e. the weakness while standing).

After two weeks she felt remarkably better and was better able to walk for longer distances, and she was kept on the same herbs. She was advised to reduce the dosage of Backbone if she started feeling hot, because, in my experience, Lupus patients and perhaps all autoimmune patients can swing rapidly between Hot and Cold conditions. In my experience, by the time lupus patients come in for herbs they no longer have butterfly patches, or other Heat signs.

Lyme Disease

Western Medicine

The first sign of Lyme disease is the appearance of a red papule on the skin 3-32 days after a tick bite. First symptoms may include fatigue, flu-like symptoms, headache, stiff neck and backache, nausea, and vomiting. Palpitations, arthritis, enlarged spleen and lymph nodes, and brain and nerve damage may occur weeks to months after disappearance of the original symptoms. Lyme disease is caused by infection by a spirochete.

Cautions

Patients with Lyme disease should be under the care of a medical doctor, particularly one who has experience treating Lyme disease.

TCM Syndromes

I am unaware of any Chinese literature concerning Lyme disease.

Chinese Herbal Therapy

We have had success using a combination of Isatis Gold and

Clear Heat
Clear Heat Clean Toxin Formula

Ingredients

English	pinyin
Isatis Extract	Ban Lan Gen and Da Qing Ye
Oldenlandia	Bai Hua She She Cao
Lonicera	Jin Yin Hua
Prunella	Xia Ku Cao
Andrographis	Chuan Xin Lian
Laminaria	Kun Bu
Viola	Zi Hua Di Ding
Cordyceps	Dong Chong Xia Cao
Licorice	Gan Cao

(see also: Istais Gold, AC-Q, Schizandra Dreams, Antler 8, Aquilaria 22, Artestatin)

Clear Heat in the initial stages of Lyme disease, usually using a high dose of two to three tablets of each formula every four hours. AC-Q formula is particularly good when treating the pain associated with

Lyme disease, as several of the ingredients have detoxicant properties. For anxiety and nerve damage we are experimenting with Schizandra Dreams, which calms the Shen and contains Kava, which was used for the treatment of syphilis before the advent of antibiotics. Syphilis and Lyme disease are both caused by spirochetes. Colostroplex, a specially prepared bovine colostrom product, can be used to treat lowered immunity and may help to rid the body of Lyme's spirochete.

Another formula that may be useful is Antler 8; some naturopathic researchers consider deer antler to be an antidote to Lyme disease. Deer antler alone may also be ordered from Chinatown herb shops. We are also experimenting with Aquilaria 22 and Artestatin in combination to help expel spirochetes that are killed off by antibiotics. If symptoms return a patient can have a much worse attack. In killing off the spirochetes, often through i.v. antibiotics, bad reactions are noticed when the spirochetes attack the heart mitochondria as well as the nerve cells.

Case Study

Mrs. Torres had been diagnosed with Lyme's disease for over one year. She was having a relapse and so her physician prescribed antibiotics. In addition she was treated with acupuncture, Colostroplex, and AC-Q. She reported much less fatigue, muscle and joint pain since taking the herbs and getting acupuncture treatments.

Menopause

Western Medicine

Menopause usually occurs around age fifty, but may begin at any time after age forty. The main symptoms are hot flashes, headache, depression, breathing difficulties, and heart palpitations. Menopause usually lasts about five years. Standard therapy involves estrogen and progesterone. Estrogen may cause fluid retention and may increase the severity of asthma, heart disorders, kidney stones, epilepsy, or migraine headaches. Estrogen combined with progesterone reduces the risk of uterine cancer that occurs with estrogen alone.

Premature menopause may be due to underlying pathologies, and is sometimes the first indication of an autoimmune disorder or diabetes. Thus any patient experiencing this should receive a thorough medical workup.

TCM Syndromes

Menopause usually involves Kidney Yin and Yang deficiency, with rising Heat. stagnant Liver Qi may be present.

Chinese Herbal Therapy

Two Immortals is an excellent choice for Kidney and Yin deficiency with rising Heat. If Two Immortals does not fully alleviate hot flashes, combine with Flavonex, which contains Kidney tonics and circulatory herbs that are rich in bioflavonoids. If Heat signs are severe, use Coptis Purge Fire. If stagnant Liver Qi predominates, Woman's Balance may be used; use only two tablets BID every other day for the first two weeks to prevent Bupleurum reaction. Two Immortals is based on Wheat Jujube decoction and another formula successfully used at Shanghai TCM Hospital. The wheat has been removed because wheat sensitivity is common in American patients.

Other Considerations

Avoid dairy products and reduce other animal products. Sugar and alcohol can also trigger hot flashes. Also useful: 400-800 IU vitamin E; Black Cohosh 1800 mg per day minimum.

Case Studies
Case 1

A thirty-five year-old woman with classical menopausal symptoms was administered the Two Immortals formula which made her symptoms go away; however she was alarmed that she started menstruating again.

Analysis: The fact that this patient started menstruating suggests that her premature menopause was due to a mild imbalance rather than a serious underlying condition. She was encouraged to continue taking the Two Immortals.

Within the same week two practitioners, one in Chicago, the other in Maine, called to say their menopausal patients had made progress initially on Two Immortals, but that their hot flashes had returned. I asked each of them if the patients were continuing to take Two Immortals. In one case, the patient had stopped taking Two Immortals one month before. I explained that since Two Immortals supplements both Yin and Yang it is a very safe and beneficial formula to take long-term, even for a year or two. Because a formula may lose some effectiveness with long-term use as a patient becomes adapted to it, administer alternate prepared formulas, such as Astra Essence, for a month every six months or so. I would only

Two Immortals
Damiana & Gotu Kola Formula

Ingredients

English	Latin/*pinyin*
Schizandra	Wu Wei Zi
Oyster shell	Mu Li
Epimedium	Yin Yang Huo
Morinda	Ba Ji Tian
Tang-kuei	Dang Gui
Ligustrum	Nu Zhen Zi
Eclipta	Han Lian Cao
Damiana	Folium Turnerae Aphrodisiacae
Gotu Kola	Radix Hydrocotyle Asiaticae
Pseudostellaria	Tai Zi Shen
Red dates	Da Zao
Anemarrhena	Zhi Mu
Phellodendron	Huang Bai
Baked Licorice	Zhi Gan Cao
Scrophularia	Xuan Shen
Eight Moon Fruit	Ba Yue Zhu

(see also: Flavonex, Coptis Purge Fire)

do this on an experimental basis; if the symptoms come back while on the Astra Essence, immediately switch back to the original formula.

Case 2

This case was more complicated. The patient was taking Flavonex in addition to Two Immortals. This is necessary in 10-20% of cases to control hot flashes. Flavonex is rich in bioflavonoids, which are used in naturopathic medicine for hot flashes, and the herbs in Flavonex astringe Kidney Essence. The combination of Two Immortals and Flavonex seems 95% effective; however this second patient was one of the other 5%.

I suggested using Coptis Purge Fire, which contains stronger Fire clearing therapy. The patient took three Two Immortals and two Coptis Purge Fire three times daily, with satisfactory results.

Analysis: Coptis Purge Fire is not routinely recommended with hot flashes since most women of menopausal age require more tonification rather than reduction therapy.

Case 3

A practitioner came up to me at a conference and said she was suffering from menopausal symptoms, with excessive anger. She was skeptical that Two Immortals could do anything (she was primarily an acupuncturist, and didn't practice herbalism). After a lengthy conversation, she decided to try one bottle even though I suggested she get two bottles, since it usually takes two bottles at the regular dosage to see any response. The next day she came back and looked like a different person; she was a lot less angry, and lighter on her feet. "Two Immortals is fantastic," she declared, and then bought four more bottles.

Analysis: As mentioned earlier, patients usually take longer to respond to tonic formulas such as Two Immortals; however, patients who do not use herbs are generally more sensitive than those who take herbs on a regular basis. One patient once called and reported insomnia after taking only one or two tablets of Astra 8, a formula without stimulants that tonifies Spleen and Lung Qi. Patients new to herbs may get a psychological boost from them, or conversely blame the herbs for any unpleasant symptoms that may be unrelated to the herbal therapy. Patients may also eat improperly or contract a flu and blame the herbs for their condition.

Menstrual Pain (Dysmenorrhea)

Western Medicine

This is the greatest cause of absence from school and work among women of menstrual age. Secondary dysmenorrhea is associated with pelvic inflammatory disease, endometriosis, use of an IUD or fertility problems. Oral contraceptives, aspirin, mefenamic acid, ibuprofen and naproxen are used to lessen the symptoms.

TCM

Dysmenorrhea is usually due to Blood stagnation with Cold signs, although it may accompany Damp Heat as well.

Crampbark Plus
Stagnant Xue Formula

Ingredients

English	Latin/*pinyin*
Crampbark	Viburnum opulis
Cinnamon twig	Gui Zhi
Achyranthes	Niu Xi
Red Peony	Chi Shao
Moutan	Mu Dan Pi
Leonurus	Yi Mu Cao
Corydalis	Yan Hu Suo
Tang-kuei	Dang Gui
Persica	Tao Ren
Zedoria	E Zhu
Sparganeum	San Leng
Cyperus	Xiang Fu
Saussurea	Mu Xiang
Carthamus	Hong Hua

(see also: Eight Treasures, Power Mushrooms, Unlocking)

Chinese Herbal Therapy

Crampbark, also known as Black Haw, is a superb antispasmodic. It is combined with warming and blood vitalizing herbs to make up Crampbark Plus. This formula is used for Cold signs and three tablets are usually taken every two hours during the onset of the cramps, although for best results it may be taken one day before the patient normally gets cramps, three tablets TID. After menstruation, patients should take Eight Treasures in order to build up Qi and Blood. If there are Heat signs, Unlocking is recommended to treat Damp Heat, Stagnant

Qi and Blood. Unlocking is taken for several months because Damp Heat has usually taken a long time to develop.

Case Study

A fisherwoman had constant terrible pains in the uterine area. She had been through intensive medical exams and was told she did not have cancer or endometriosis. When I asked if a hot water bottle improved the pain, I was told she was never without it. She also had pale skin and a pale tongue.

She was put on Crampbark Plus, at least three tablets TID, with an additional three tablets if the pain resumed, and two tablets of Power Mushrooms TID. Within five days the woman reported that she was 90% better. I suggested maintaining the herbs for several more weeks.

Analysis: After determining this was a Cold condition (her profession created situations very similar to those seen in China where the uterus is exposed to cold while working in the fields), I felt she needed Crampbark Plus to warm up her uterus and activate Blood, and also Power Mushrooms as a general tonic.

Multiple Sclerosis

Western Medicine

MS is a progressive disease of the central nervous system. Exercise and staying busy are valuable in causing a remission in symptoms. Physical therapy is often helpful. At this time there is no Western cure, however a healthy immune system is extremely important. For more information contact the Multiple Sclerosis Society at 1-212-986-3240.

One suspected, although not proven, cause of MS is an autoimmune reaction. For this reason, the German government says echinacea and other immune stimulants are contraindicated in MS.

Power Mushrooms

Ganoderma, Shiitake, Tremella

Ingredients

English	Latin/*pinyin*
Ganoderma (Rei Shi)	Ling Zhi
Shiitake (Lentinin)	Lentinus edodes
Tremella	Bai Mu Er
Poria	Fu Ling
Polyporus	Zhu Ling

(see also: Phellostatin, Marrow Plus, Backbone, Nine Flavor Tea, Heavenly Water, Coptis Purge Fire, Water's Way, Temper Fire)

TCM

The first stage involves Lung Heat. In the second stage there is Kidney and Liver deficiency, and excess Damp Heat. Blood stagnation must also be addressed.

Chinese Herbal Therapy

Power Mushrooms combines herbs that regulate an immune system that is over-functioning or under-functioning, on the basis of Japanese research. Ganoderma, shiitake, tremella, polyporus and poria dry Dampness. The formula usually gives clients more energy. If there is Damp Heat, Phellostatin may be used to rid the body of Damp Heat and tonify the Spleen. This can be combined with Coptis Purge Fire, or Water's Way for additional drying.

For later stage MS, Marrow Plus is helpful for vitalizing and tonifying the Blood. Temper Fire (Zhi Bai Di Huang Wan) may be used for Kidney Yin deficiency and deficient Heat.

Case Study

A man in his early forties diagnosed with MS, with wasting paralysis, weak tingling of the legs, a purplish tongue with yellow coating in the back, and occasional fits of rage, came in for herbal therapy. He was taking Symmatril, an antiviral drug which helped his fatigue greatly.

I suggested two tablets of Backbone, one tablet of Nine Flavor Tea, and two tablets of Heavenly Water TID. Backbone, which regenerates Kidney Yang and activates Blood, was given to try to treat the paralysis. Nine Flavor Tea was used to counter the potentially overheating effects of Backbone, and Heavenly Water was used to treat Liver Qi stagnation as evidenced by the rage, and also to tonify the Spleen and ventilate Heat through the Lung.

The client reported he felt calmer and stronger three weeks after taking the herbs.

Obesity

Western Medicine

Those who are twenty percent or more over normal weight for their age, build, and height are considered to have excess body fat. These individuals are at risk for cardiovascular disease, diabetes, high blood pressure, kidney disorders, liver damage, pregnancy complications, and psychological distress. Developing sustainable healthy eating habits is far more important than short-term dieting. Deprivation also does not usually work, because it often leads to re-bound eating, i.e. eating only carrot sticks at the party may lead to eating a carton of ice cream later as a reward. A deprivation diet may also alter the body metabolism, so it is more difficult to lose weight or to prevent regaining lost pounds.

Astra 18 Diet

Ingredients

English	pinyin
Astragalus	Huang Qi
Alisma	Ze Xie
Gardenia	Zhi Zi
Cyperus	Xiang Fu
Stephania	Fang Ji
Citrus	Chen Pi
Tang kuei	Dang Gui
Sargassum	Hai Zao
Laminaria	Kun Bu
White Attractylodes	Bai Zhu
Scute	Huang Qin
Siler	Fang Feng
Magnolia	Hou Po
Ginger	Gan Jiang
Pinellia	Ban Xia
Red Peony	Chi Shao
Platycodon	Jie Geng
Licorice	Gan Cao

(see also: GB-6, Stomach Tabs, Quiet Digestion, Astra Diet Tea, Woman's Balance, Heavenly Water)

TCM

Dampness, Phlegm accumulation, Qi deficiency, Heat, food stagnation

Chinese Herbal Therapy

Modern Western research validates the principals of Chinese dietary therapy (see also: Chinese Dietary Therapy). Eating regularly, regular exercise (not to exhaustion), and drinking tea instead of coffee, soda, and milk are also important. Artificial sweeteners may increase appetite, and lead to weight gain. It is important to treat the individual signs and symptoms. Patients undergoing rapid weight loss may help to prevent gallbladder stones by taking GB-6. Women who have premenstrual cravings may take Woman's Balance or Heavenly Water. Individuals who are obese and have sluggish digestion should take Quiet Digestion along with making dietary modifications. Patients who are obese and have manifestations of Phlegm can usually benefit from Stomach Tabs. Astra 18 Diet, a broad-spectrum formula, is designed to clear Dampness and Phlegm, disperse stagnant Qi, and tonify Spleen Qi. It is recommended along with Astra Diet Tea or other sweet tasting teas as a dessert substitute.

Case study

A thirty-five year-old woman, with a long history of binge diets and severe PMS, came to me. Her tongue was pale, and her pulse was weak despite a robust appearance. She was fifteen pounds overweight. I suggested that she eat three meals a day and cut out her fruit juice fasting, substituting simple meals of rice and vegetables, soups and whole fruits. Since she was already taking several nutritional supplements, I suggested she take two tablets of Woman's Balance TID. She also began a rigorous aerobics program. Within six weeks she reported that she lost ten pounds, and was feeling much more balanced.

Analysis: Fruit juices, even the unsweetened varieties, contain too much concentrated sugar, and should not be taken as a meal replacement. They cause Dampness which leads to Qi stagnation. In this case the stagnant Qi explained the severe PMS, and therefore the recommendation to use Woman's Balance.

Parasitic Infection

Western Medicine

There is a growing presence of parasitic infection in the West. Parasitic infection may be present in patients with acute digestive disorders, and symptoms similar to chronic fatigue syndrome (CFIDS), especially if they have visited Third World countries or have drunk untreated water while camping. Common parasitic infections include giardia, *Entameba histolytica,* and *Blastocystis hominis.* Parasitic symptoms may mimic CFIDS, and that there is a common factor of weakened immunity in CFIDS, candidiasis, and parasitic infection. Standard medical treatment involves Flagyl and other antiparasitic drugs.

TCM

TCM strategies include Clear Summer Heat, Purge Parasites, and Tonify Spleen.

Chinese Herbal Therapy

Chinese herbal therapy can be effective against these infections, but prolonged therapy is necessary. The formulas should be administered one month longer than a test shows the clearing of the parasites. Artestatin is a Clear Summer Heat formula which contains Artemisia annua (Qing Hao). It has been used with success for Malaria, and with some success for Giardia. The formula contains Dichroa, which is antiparasitic, Brucea, which is said to destroy amoebas in the cyst stage, Dolichos and Pulsatilla, which are antiparasitic, and Coptis, which is anti-microbial. The remaining herbs in the formula tonify the Spleen. This formula is used primarily to treat diarrhea and parasites that are specifically amoebic. Aquilaria 22 is a broad spectrum formula comprised of half antiparasitic agents and half Spleen tonics. It treats constipation and can be used for parasitic infections of unknown origin, liver flukes, and pinworms, since many of the herbs also expel these pathogens. In severe cases the two formulas may be combined. It is generally recommended that Artestatin be followed up with Aquilaria 22 after approximately three months.

Quiet Digestion is a useful adjunct formula for the acute abdominal symptoms. Follow directions on the label. In severe cases the Bioradiance formula may also be administered. Many of the ingredients in this formula have been used traditionally.

Notes

Follow TCM diet. Western therapy using grapefruit seed extract is helpful; however it is very cooling and must be balanced with other herbs. It is an excellent adjunct to Artestatin.

Case Study

A woman in her mid-thirties who sought my help was infected with *Blastocystis hominis*, cryptosporidium and candida. She was also experiencing food allergies and a worsening of menstrual cramps and PMS.

Her tongue was red in the

Artestatin
Artemisia Annua Concentrate Formula

Ingredients

English	*pinyin*
Artemisia annua	Qing Hao
Dichroa	Shu Chi
Pulsatilla	Bai Tou Weng
Magnolia bark	Hou Po
Pinellia	Ban Xia
Pogostemon	Huo Xiang
Dolichos	Bai Bian Dou
Ginseng	Ren Shen
Citrus	Chen Pi
Licorice	Gan Cao
Coptis	Huang Lian
Red Atractylodes	Cang Zhu
Ginger	Gan Jiang
Cardamon	Sha Ren

(see also: Aquilaria 22, Quiet Digestion, Bioradiance)

Liver and Gallbladder areas, and she had a chronic low-grade fever. She also had vaginal itching and abdominal bloating, so I recommended GB-6 for Gallbladder Heat. I also recommended Aquilaria 22, since she had chronic constipation. Woman's Balance was given to her ten days before her period began, to help alleviate PMS and menstrual cramps. Finally I told her to take Crampbark Plus only if there were menstrual cramps.

The patient found her constipation was alleviated after two to three weeks. She also had significantly less PMS and menstrual cramps, although she did have to take the Crampbark Plus three times, at three tablets per dose. When I consulted with her about six weeks later she was having some diarrhea, and so I suggested adding Artestatin. Using Aquilaria 22 with Artestatin provides broad spectrum action. I suggested she discontinue GB-6. The patient was very happy with the progress she made.

Analysis: A previous practitioner had recommended a Kidney Yin tonic which did not help her condition and might have made her Spleen more Damp, therefore she sought out my services. Obviously, this practitioner got confused between Damp Heat signs and Yin deficiency signs. This is a common mistake. In a Damp Heat condition the patient has a sense of constant fever, whereas the Yin deficient patient will have only afternoon or evening fevers. Damp Heat in the Liver and Gallbladder will cause a bitter taste in the mouth, although I find it rare that American patients complain of a bitter taste unless they have a lot of sour regurgitation.

Pediatrics

Acute Cold and Flu Treatment: Isatis Gold, Yin Chao Jin

Flu and Infection Prevention: Astra C, Prosperous Farmer

Phlegm: Lucid Channel, Stomach Tabs

Bedwetting: Astra Essence

Raspy Cough: Wise Judge

Hyperactivity: Ease Plus

Acne: Colorful Phoenix

Diaper Rash: Vagistatin (applied topically)

Administration

The best method is to swallow the tablets directly. If this is not possible, tablets may be ground and added to applesauce, peanut butter or honey. The tablets may also be ground to a powder and added to boiling water to make a tea. This can be sweetened or followed by a glass of fruit juice. The tea may also be squirted in the mouth with a dropper. With K'an tinctures use 1/8 dropper to 8 oz of grape juice, or fill the rest of the dropper with warm water and squirt into the child's mouth. Droppers should be squirted as far as possi-

Astra C	
Ingredients	
English	*pinyin*
Ascorbic Acid (Vitamin C)	
Astragalus	Huang Qi
White Atractylodes	Bai Zhu
Siler	Fang Feng
Zinc Citrate	
Rose Hips	
Acerola	

ble at the back of the tongue, which is less sensitive than the front of the tongue. With Vagistatin, take the capsule apart, mix with a small amount of water and apply topically.

Dosage

The adult dosage is 3 tablets or 1/4 dropper of K'an extracts TID. Some practitioners recommend lower dosages for children; others recommend the adult dosage for children over the age of five. Children progress through illness quickly because they generally have strong Yang Qi.

Case Studies

Diaper Rash

A baby had diaper rash. Diaper rash is often due to candida infection. I told the practitioner to empty Vagistatin capsules and make a paste, to be kept on as long as possible. The mother called back the following day and reported that the rash had improved 50% overnight.

Cough

A five year-old boy had been coughing about every ten seconds for the past few days, getting little sleep. At night his cough was productive with clear phlegm; during the day it was dry and barking. Despite the coughing his overall energy was good.

I suggested using two tablets of Wise Judge every few hours during the day to help soothe the dryness, help slide off phlegm stuck to his throat, and Lucid Channel to resolve Phlegm. I suggested using two tablets each of Minor Blue Dragon and Lucid Channel at bedtime to treat the productive cough. Two days later I saw him and his cough had completely disappeared. As a follow-up, Astra 8 was recommended to build up Spleen, Lung, and Wei Qi.

Fever With Cough

A four year-old boy was running a temperature of 104 degrees. His dad, a practitioner, administered four tablets of Coptis Purge Fire and three tablets of Isatis Gold, in two doses, taken as teas with honey. Four hours later the boy broke out into a sweat. Shortly after that, the fever came down.

On the second day he was given Clear Air and Isatis Gold, two tablets of each as tea with honey, throughout the day for his cough. On day three he was able to go to school, and he was taking the Isatis Gold and Clear Air before and after school.

He developed a barking cough on day four and the Wise Judge formula was used. After three days the cough disappeared.

Analysis: In this case the formula changed every day, unlike that for an adult, who would often progress more slowly.

Allergies with Hives

A twelve year-old boy with multiple allergies frequently broke out in hives. His practitioner got very good results with Xanthium Relieve Surface. He administered three tablets TID, which is the adult dose. As long as the child is on the herbal formula the hives do not occur. He also takes Astra Isatis, one tablet TID, to tonify his immune system to keep the hives from reoccurring.

Postpartum

Western Medicine

After childbirth there may be irritability, fatigue, and loss of appetite.

TCM

Qi and Blood deficiency. There also may be Blood stasis.

Postpartum
Qi and Jing Formula

Ingredients

English	pinyin
Ginseng	Ren Shen
Astragalus	Huang Qi
Rehmannia	Shu Di Huang
Salvia	Dan Shen
Poria	Fu Ling
Leonurus	Yi Mu Cao
Tang-kuei	Dang Gui
White Peony	Bai Shao
Ho-shou-wu	He Shou Wu
Ligusticum	Chuan Xiong
Gelatinum	E Jiao
Crataegus	Shan Zha
Rubia	Qian Cao Gen
Citrus	Chen Pi
Artemesia	Ai Ye
Licorice	Gan Cao
Atractylodes	Bai Zhu

(see also: Astra Essence)

Chinese Herbal Therapy

The postpartum formula was developed by Jake Fratkin, OMD, LAc, and successfully used in his clinic. In cases of difficult or long labor, combine with a Kidney tonic such as Astra Essence. This formula may be taken while nursing. Note that a nursing baby will be receiving a small dose of herbs, and therefore it is possible, although not likely, that the baby will develop constipation or diarrhea from Postpartum, in which case the dosage should be reduced.

Case Study

A young woman who had been to one of the best herbalists in San Francisco had been tired since giving birth to her third child. Her pulse was very deficient and her tongue also indicated Cold. Since the patient did not live in San Francisco and hated drinking tea, she came to me. She was relieved that she could take tablets rather than tea, since the taste was objectionable and the preparation time-consuming. I recommended Postpartum, two tablets TID, with Astra Essence, two tablets TID. After five weeks, the woman thought the tablets were much more effective than the tea she had previously taken.

Analysis: Astra Essence was included since it offers more Kidney support than Postpartum, which mainly tonifies the Spleen and Blood, and normalizes the uterus.

Premenstrual Syndrome (PMS), Postmenstrual Fatigue

Western Medicine

Signs and symptoms occur approximately ten days before the menstrual period begins. Common symptoms include anxiety, abdominal bloating, finger and ankle swelling, breast distension, depression, headache, and irritability.

TCM

Liver Qi stagnation with rising Heat; may include Spleen Qi deficiency.

Chinese Herbal Therapy

The standard Xiao Yao San formula for relaxing Liver Qi has been modified with herbs for Heat clearing and Blood moving and is called Woman's Balance (Dan Zhi Xiao Yao San). It is important that patients who have stored a lot of anger take this formula on alternate days and not exceed four tablets per day for the first week. This will avoid a lot of anger being expressed at once. Many women have Liver Qi stagnation due to Blood deficiency. In this case Eight Treasures can be started postmenstrually and Woman's Balance may be started ten days before the menstrual period begins. If the patient has Spleen Qi deficiency, Heavenly Water can be taken at the full dose since Gota Kola has been substituted for Bupleurum.

In certain cases I have had clients take Woman's Balance and Heavenly Water on alternate days with good success. This is used with angry patients with simultaneous Qi deficiency.

Notes

Diet/lifestyle modifications include stress reduction, TCM diet, vitamin B6, and regular exercise.

Case Studies

Case 1

A patient had spotting after regular periods, and symptoms of Spleen Qi deficiency, Liver Qi congestion, Kidney Qi deficiency. Her pulse was wiry, and her tongue was pale in the center and red in the Liver and Gallbladder areas. Heavenly Water is very useful for Spleen Qi deficiency and Liver Qi congeston, and has yielded good results with spotting. I suggested combining it with Astra Essence to boost the Kidney Qi. After two months she reported no more spotting, and feeling more balanced premenstrually.

Case 2

A female client in her late thirties was seen by a colleague. She had the following symptoms: severe PMS with mood swings, anger, low back pain, headaches, and feeling hot all over. Her tongue was red, and her pulse was fast and wiry during this period. She also had very painful menstrual cramps. After menstruation she felt extreme exhaustion, had a pale tongue and slow pulse.

I recommended using Eight Treasures, three tablets TID postmenstrually, and then twelve days before her period,

---

Woman's Balance
Tang-kuei Herbal Formula

Ingredients

English	*pinyin*
Bupleurum	Chai Hu
Tang-kuei	Dang Gui
White Peony	Bai Shao
Salvia	Dan Shen
Poria	Fu Ling
Atractylodes	Bai Zhu
Cyperus	Xiang Fu
Citrus	Chen Pi
Moutan	Mu Dan Pi
Gardenia	Zhi Zi
Ginger	Gan Jiang
Licorice	Gan Cao

(see also: Eight Treasures, Heavenly Water, Unlocking)

---

using a combination of Woman's Balance, one tablet TID up until menstruation, and Unlocking, three tablets TID through the end of bleeding. After three months most of the symptoms were considerably relieved.

Analysis: Premenstrually, Woman's Balance was used for Liver stagnation with Heat signs and Unlocking was used to clear Damp Heat, as well as stagnation of Qi and Blood. Postmenstrually, Eight Treasures was used to tonify Blood and Qi and warm up her Cold pattern.

Prostate Enlargement

Western Medicine

Nearly 60% of men between between forty and sixty have an enlarged prostate condition known as benign prostatic hypertrophy or hyperplasia (BPH). The percentage rises to 90% by age seventy. Symptoms include bladder obstruction, frequent urination, hesitancy, dribbling urine, and getting up at night to urinate. Standard medical treatment involves surgery. Nutritionally, zinc, pumpkin seeds (one half cup per day) may also be helpful. BPH and cancer of the prostate have symptoms in common, and anyone with prostate symptoms should receive a complete medical exam.

TCM

Kidney Yang deficiency, Damp Heat in the Lower Burner.

Chinese Herbal Therapy

Successful treatment depends upon differentiation. For acute symptoms, the Akebia Moist Heat formula, based upon Ba Zheng San, may be used. To quickly alleviate frequent urination, Astra Essence may be used; this builds up the Kidney and consolidates fluids. For long-term herbal therapy, Essence Chamber, a combination of Chinese and Western herbs, has been very successful. Saw Palmetto berries have been successfully used as a folk medicine and in clinical studies. It may also be used by any male for a few weeks a year to prevent BPH. If there is significant swelling the patient should take the formula for one to two years.

Notes

Avoid shellfish, alcohol, and fried and spicy food. According to Pritikin, elevated cholesterol levels will cause crystalline formations that settle in the prostate, and cause additional swelling. A sitz bath may be taken for ten minutes at 105 degrees, followed by cool sponging of the pelvic area. This relaxes the opening of the urinary passageway. Alternating hot and cold water is helpful.

Case Studies
Case 1

A man in his fifties had a biomedical diagnosis of benign hypertrophy of the prostate. His main symptom was getting up the night several times to urinate. I recommended a combination of Astra Essence and Essence Chamber. In my experience Astra Essence is able to reduce frequent urination rapidly, while Essence Chamber is specific for prostatic hypertrophy. He was taking two tablets of each formula TID. Within two weeks he reported that he was not needing to get up as many times at night, and therefore he was getting much better sleep. I suggested that he keep taking the formulas for at least six months, and continue to get regular medical checkups.

Case 2

A practitioner in his late fifties with BPH had to get up three and four times a night to urinate. He had tried several formulas containing Saw Palmetto, including Essence Chamber, and there was only slight improvement. I suggested he

---

Essence Chamber
Saw Palmetto Formula

Ingredients

English	Latin/*pinyin*
Patrinia	Bai Jiang Cao
Saw Palmetto	Serenoa serrulata
Salvia	Dan Shen
Vaccaria	Wang Bu Liu Xing
Liquidambar	Lu Lu Tong
Hydrangea	Hydrangea arborscentis
Damiana	Turnerae aphrodisiacae
Poria	Fu Ling
Tokoro	Bi Jie
Abutilon	Dong Gua Zi

(see also: Astra Essence, Akebia Moist Heat)

---

start taking Astra Essence, and within three days he was only getting up once per night to urinate. After six weeks taking the Astra Essence he only had to get up every other night or so to urinate. I decided to reformulate Essence Chamber and he is evaluating the new version for his BPH.

Case 3: Prostate/Vasectomy Complications

A fifty year-old man who had recently undergone a vasectomy developed an infection in the testes following the operation, with a lump where the incision was made. The patient had been given antibiotics by his medical doctor, but was not responding. I suggested a combination of Unlocking and Flavonex, two tablets of each formula QID.

After several weeks the patient's condition improved. I recommended tonification with Astra Essence to follow up the cooling effects of Unlocking.

Analysis: Vasectomies tend to cause or aggravate Qi and Blood stagnation and can cause testicular pain and swelling, as well as other conditions. Flavonex has anti-inflammatory properties due to the bioflavonoid components in the formula, and increases circulation. Importantly, Flavonex is not a particularly warming formula, which could cause a worsening of the inflammation. Unlocking is used for Qi and Blood stagnation, as well as Damp Heat in the Lower Burner.

Shoulder and Neck Tension, Whiplash, Injury

Western Medicine

Differentiation must be made between injury or post-injury and shoulder and neck tension that is brought about by stress. Proper posture while lifting or performing a repetitive motion is the most important preventive therapy. Repetitive motions must be avoided whenever possible. For example, athletes can and should cross-train, whereas it is more difficult in an occupational situation. There are excellent books available by those who teach the Alexander or Feldenkrais techniques. Physical therapy or consultation with ergonomic experts may be needed.

TCM

The Liver makes sure the Qi flows smoothly; therefore if there is repressed anger or other emotions the Qi will not flow smoothly and there will be pain and discomfort. This condition can be treated satisfactorily with Chinese herbs. The Liver also controls the sinews and tendons, whereas the Spleen controls the muscles.

If the condition is post-injury, even if the injury was several years ago, Blood stagnation must be addressed.

Chinese Herbal Therapy

SPZM is an empirical formula used in China to treat upper-body spasm and cramps and is particularly useful for whiplash and other injuries affecting the shoulder and neck. It can be used in conjunction with injury formulas such as Resinall K.

For long-standing shoulder and neck tension due to stress, I have had exceptionally good results using Ease 2, which is a traditional formula Bupleurum and Cinnamon (Chai Hu Gui Zhi Tang) with added Pueraria (Ge Gen) for shoulder and neck tension. Calm Spirit is added if there are signs of Yin deficiency, on a long-term basis, or on a short-term basis to augment Ease 2. If the patient has a weak

Spleen and/or loose stools, Calm Spirit should only be used short-term, or combined with a Spleen tonic such as Six Gentlemen or Quiet Digestion which counter the Dampening effect of Calm Spirit, which contains mostly Yin and Blood tonics, but also contains enzymes to intercept free radicals that can accompany stress.

Ease 2 is also successfully used in order to help "hold" chiropractic adjustments.

Case Studies
Case 1
A patient taking fifty vitamin pills a day came in with shoulder and neck tension, dry throat, irritability, and anxiety. The tongue was purple, not coated, and the pulse was wiry. The patient had extreme shoulder and neck tension; therefore I put the patient on Ease 2, three tablets TID, and Calm Spirit, three tablets TID, with the suggestion that the patient take up yoga or similar stretching exercises and cut down some of the vitamins.

This patient was reluctant to cut down vitamins and decided to combine them with the herbs. The patient was immune-compromised and had frequent colds, which is why he was on so many supplements. Most of these were prescribed by a nutritionally-oriented doctor.

Ease 2
Bupleurum & Cinnamon Combination

Ingredients

English	pinyin
Bupleurum	Chai Hu
Pueraria	Ge Gen
Pinellia	Ban Xia
Cinnamon	Gui Zhi
Peony	Bai Shao
Ginseng	Ren Shen
Scute	Huang Qui
Licorice	Gan Cao
Ginger	Gan Jiang

(see also: Calm Spirit)

The patient found immediate symptomatic relief with the Ease 2 and Calm Spirit formulas, which I have found to work well together. The patient reported that the herbs seemed to take only about an hour to be effective, but that the pain crept back after a few hours. Patient was quite "amazed at how relaxed" the herbs made him feel.

The patient did not drink alcohol but was a coffee drinker. I suggested on the follow-up he reduce or eliminate the amino acids and CO-Q-10, which I guessed were more warming than the basic vitamins and minerals.

After cutting down these supplements the patient was less irritable and had considerably less shoulder and neck tension. I suggested he maintain the herbs for another two weeks (it had been four weeks) and phase out the Calm Spirit except for the mornings, when his shoulder and neck tension were worse, and continue taking the Ease 2.

Analysis: Certain vitamins and certain amino acids and other metabolites can be very warming. My guess is they boost the Yang Qi and overheat a congested liver.

Case 2

A small woman in her thirties came in complaining of extended colds and flu, constant shoulder and neck tension, gastroenteritis, and excess stress. Her tongue was pale, and her pulse faint. Not only did she get constant colds and flus, but it usually took her two to three weeks to recover from them, at which point she usually got another cold or flu shortly after, indicating weak Wei Qi. I suggested Ease 2, three tablets TID, since this formula treats shoulder, neck, and upper body tension. It also harmonizes the interior and exterior. I suggested she also take Astra C, to build up her Wei Qi (defensive energy), at least two tablets TID. This formula also contains zinc, which is an immune builder. I suggested that she discontinue taking these formulas when coming down with a cold or flu, and take the Isatis Gold formula, three tablets every few hours. If the cold or flu lingered I said it was okay to start taking the Ease 2 if her shoulder and neck symptoms returned, but that she should not take Astra C until a week after a cold or flu, as this could trap invading virus or bacteria.

I decided not to treat the gastrointestinal complaints at this time, as the patient did not have enough money to take additional formulas, and shoulder/neck tension was her primary concern. In addition, the Ease 2 helps dry Dampness and tonify the Spleen, and thus aids in digestion.

Sinus Infections

Western Medicine

Sinus infection is usually treated with repeated courses of antibiotics. Western drugs may mask the true signs and symptoms, so it may be necessary to ascertain what the color of the phlegm was before any medication was started. Prior use of Western drugs almost always necessitates the use of tonic herbs.

Nasal Tabs
Pueraria Combination

Ingredients

English	pinyin
Ma-Huang	Ma Huang
Magnolia	Xin Yi
Pueraria	Ge Gen
Rhubarb	Da Huang
Coix	Yi Yi Ren
Gypsum	Shi Gao
Cinnamon twig	Gui Zhi
Peony	Bai Shao
Ginger	Gan Jiang
Licorice	Gan Cao
Ligusticum	Chuan Xiong
Jujube	Da Zao
Platycodon	Jie Geng

(see also: Isatis Gold, Minor Blue Dragon, Six Gentlemen, Quiet Digestion, Ginseng & Gecko, Phellostatin, Lucid Channel)

TCM Syndromes

It is important to differentiate the color of the phlegm. White or clear indicates Cold. Yellow or colored indicates Heat. Usually, repeated sinus infections are due to long-term deficiency of Kidney, Lung, or Spleen.

Chinese Herbal Therapy

For sinus infections in the acute stage, use Nasal Tabs, which directs the action to the head, coupled with Isatis Gold, which has antibiotic properties. This protocol is suitable for yellow or colored phlegm. If there is copious clear or white phlegm, Minor Blue Dragon coupled with Six Gentlemen is recommended. Particularly if the tongue has a greasy coat, Quiet Digestion is often very useful, as the root of sinus infections is Dampness and Phlegm in the Spleen.

To prevent recurrence, the Ginseng and Gecko formula may be applied if there is wheezing or asthma. It is not appropriate in the acute stage of asthma (see Asthma). Use this formula for several months. If there is no wheezing, apply Quiet Digestion for one month; then tonify with Six Gentlemen or Astra 8 for several months.

Phellostatin may be used in cases of long-term yellow discharge, as this formula rids the body of Damp Heat in the Intestines and tonifies the Spleen. This is particularly important if the patient has signs and symptoms of candidiasis, and also has Heat-related digestive disorders. Since many patients with frequent sinus infections have taken long-term antibiotic prescriptions, always suspect candidiasis. For postnasal drip Lucid Channel is recommended.

Case Study

A fifteen year-old boy with chronically stuffed sinuses, a propensity for getting sinus infections, and a cough with difficulty breathing, responded well to the following protocol: Nasal Tabs for opening up the sinuses, and Ginseng and Gecko as a constitutional formula. He takes the adult dose of Ginseng and Gecko, three tablets TID, and he takes Nasal Tabs as needed.

Analysis: Some advanced practitioners consider allergic rhinitis and sinusitis to respond well to Kidney Yang tonification as part of the treatment. Ginseng and Gecko may be used with Dampness and Qi deficiency. In this case Ginseng and Gecko is used to strengthen the Lung, which in turn is said to keep the nose open. This young man reported less nasal stuffiness and coughing by using the two formulas.

Skin Disorders (Dermatology)

Western Medicine

Select skin diseases respond very favorably to Chinese herbal medicine, but others respond only under the supervision of a master herbalist, who can prescribe oral as well as topical herbs, changing the prescription on a weekly basis as needed. In my experience psoriasis is such a case. Stubborn tinea cannot be treated satisfactorily with Chinese herbs, while mild cases may respond to Chinese herbs or to tea tree oil. I have gotten very favorable results with certain cases of acne, hives, poison ivy, poison oak, herpes zoster, and herpes simplex (see Herpes), ringworm, crabs, impetigo, and Kaposi's sarcoma. Practitioners who have not had much experience may want to try suggestions in this book before referring to an experienced herbalist.

TCM

Many conditions are considered Wind Heat conditions. Yin deficiency and Damp Heat may also be involved. Aromatic constituents may eliminate certain microorganisms. For more information consult Nissi Wang's book on dermatology, to be published by Eastland Press.

Chinese Herbal Therapy

I have successfully used Xanthium Relieve Surface in the treatment of hives, poison ivy, and poison oak. The dosage is usually three tablets every two to three hours until there is a reduction of symptoms. If no symptomatic results are seen, use one tablet of Astra C for each three tablets of Xanthium Relieve Surface. For ringworm and crabs I have made Cir-Q into a topical application by crushing up two tablets, adding boiling water (about 8 oz. per two tablets), and letting the mixture soak overnight in a refrigerator. The result is a very dark liquid that can be dabbed onto the affected area several times a day. When the liquid runs out, repeat the recipe. CIR-Q contains strong aromatics that in one case of crabs was totally effective within three days. In a case of scabies it was effective within ten days (in conjunction with a naturopathic remedy). It was also effective, combined with another remedy, in a case of ringworm.

There have been good reports using Zedoaria Tablets with the initial stages of Kaposi's sarcoma. Another new formula that can be tried for Kaposi's sarcoma is Eupolyphaga Tablets. Resinall K has been used successfully in two cases of impetigo, when used topically every few hours. It has also been used with varying degrees of success topically for skin fungal infections including athletes foot.

Case Studies

Case 1

A seventeen year-old man who was very active athletically had acne, with a rapid pulse and a dry red tongue. Within four days of taking Nine Flavor Tea, three tablets TID, he had a significant reduction in acne. Within two weeks his acne almost disappeared.

Xanthium Relieve Surface

Ingredients

English	pinyin
Xanthium	Cang Er Zi
Chrysanthemum	Ju Hua
Astragalus	Huang Qi
Ligusticum	Chuan Xiong
Schizonepeta	Jing Jie
Phellodendron	Huang Bai
Siler	Fang Feng
Angelica	Bai Zhi
Rehmannia	Shu Di Huang
Mume	Wu Mei
Platycodon	Jie Geng
Asarum	Xi Xin
Anemarrhena	Zhi Mu
Licorice	Gan Cao

(see also: Cir-Q, Nine Flavor Tea, Phellostatin, Zedoaria Tablets, Resinall K)

Case 2

Another case of acne was a twenty-eight year-old man with a pale tongue with a greasy yellow coating, a submerged pulse, a history of irritable bowel syndrome, and a fondness for sweets, coffee drinking, and smoking. He said that his acne had worsened since moving to the Pacific northwest, which has a cold, damp climate. His acne was reduced after about two months of taking Phellostatin, three tablets TID, acidophilus, and a reduction in sweets (including fruit juices), and using special skin care cosmetics that did not contain allergens.

Case 3

A patient with extensive ringworm was anxious to try herbs rather than drugs. Having received excellent results in treating scabies using Cir-Q with two patients and medium results with a third patient with a lot of psychological complaints, I instructed the patient to apply it topically every two hours, alternating with Resinall K applied topically. Resinall K, being an extract, is already in liquid form and easier to apply if the patient is not at home. Within a few days the patient reported that the ringworm was gone.

Case 4

A patient with cystic acne who had been on antibiotics for four months came in. He had a fast pulse and red tongue with a yellow coat. He was put on Clear Heat — it was suggested that he take six tablets initially and then take four tablets every three hours. Within three days the acne dried up.

Analysis: Often acne is due to excess Heat. This patient had obvious Heat signs. Resinall K is startlingly effective for some skin conditions and ineffective for others. It contains mostly Blood activating herbs, some of which have been useful in treating skin conditions. We have had good results using Resinall K with stubborn foot fungus, impetigo, and an undiagnosed facial fungus where a colleague was told by her patient "If you clear this up I'll give you a million dollars." The condition cleared up within three weeks after applying Resinall K twice daily. The last time I talked to her, the colleague had yet to collect the million dollars.

Stress and Anxiety, Insomnia, Depression, Emotional Stress

Western Medicine

Most people can cope with short-term stress, but long-term stress can have serious health consequences. Irritability, high blood pressure, headaches, neck aches, diarrhea, and loss of appetite are caused by stress. Digestive disorders and depression can also be caused by stress. Our body prepares for stress associated with "fight or flight." Thus the heart rate increases, fats and sugars are released from reserve supplies, the blood prepares for clotting, and the digestive system shuts down. The adrenal medulla secretes adrenaline and other stress-related hormones.

TCM

If the mind is disturbed from emotional upsets, there will be exhaustion of Blood or Yin. Blood and Yin deficiency can also lead to emotional upset. Heart Yin deficiency is characterized by insomnia, anxiety, low grade fever especially in the afternoon, night sweating, dry mouth and throat, and Heat in the extremities. A related condition, Heart Blood deficiency, has many of the same characteristics. However, a patient with Heart Blood deficiency finds it difficult to fall asleep, though once asleep he or she will sleep well. A Heart Yin deficient patient will find it difficult to fall asleep and will wake up several times during the night.

Liver Qi stagnation is characterized by shoulder and neck tension, depression, melancholy, bitter taste in the mouth, nausea, sour regurgitation, belching, abdominal distention, diarrhea, PMS, irregular and/or painful periods, chest distention, lump in the throat, and difficulty swallowing. Whereas Liver Qi stagnation is caused by frustration and anger, Heart Yin and Blood deficiencies are usually due to anxiety, worry, and life on the run.

Chinese Herbal Therapy

Calm Spirit is a special formula that nourishes Blood and Heart Yin, with Peony to help with Liver Qi stagnation. It is a modification of Ding Xin Wan, a traditional formula, with magnesium, taurine and enzymes for quick results. Excellent results can be obtained combining Calm Spirit with Ease 2 or Ease Plus.

Liver Qi stagnation is treated with Ease 2. This is the traditional formula Bupleurum and Cinnamon (Chai Hu Gui Zhi Tang) modified with Pueraria (Ge Gen). This formula treats shoulder and neck tension, and is indicated for the patient with loose stools. In this situation there are generally signs of Cold and weakness.

Ease Plus, based on the traditional formula Bupleurum and Dragonbone (Chai Hu Jia Long Gu Mu Li Tang), is more appropriate for Liver Qi stagnation with constipation. In this presentation there are usually signs of Heat and greater strength, and the pulse would be more forceful. The patient may have stress and anxiety if an addictive substance has been withdrawn, and is generally angry.

Woman's Balance, based on the traditional formula Dan Zhi Xiao Yao San (a combination of Bupleurum and Tang-kuei formula and Bupleurum and Peony formula) is useful for women or men with Liver Qi stagnation with rising Heat.

Calm Spirit
Modified Ding Xin Wan

Ingredients

Enzymes:	derived from:
Peroxidase	Horseradish root
Catalase	Aspergillus niger
Amylase	Aspergillus oryzae
Protease	Aspergillus oryzae
Lipase	Aspergillus oryzae

Herbs:	
English	*pinyin*
Biota	Bai Zi Ren
Tang-kuei	Dang Gui
Fu-shen	Fu Shen
Polygala	Yuan Zhi
Zizyphus	Suan Zao Ren
Peony	Bai Shao
Ophiopogon	Mai Men Dong
Codonopsis	Dang Shen
Succinum	Hu Po

Also contains:

Taurine
Magnesium aspartate

(see also: Ease 2, Eash Plus, Woman's Balance, Shen-Gem, Aspiration)

For Heart Blood deficiency, Shen-Gem, based on the traditional formula Gui Pi Tang, with additional relaxant Amber (Ho Po) and Salvia (Dan Shen) to circulate the blood, is usually used for anxiety, insomnia, and stress due to deficiency characterized by pale complexion, cold extremities, and fatigue. In my experience this formula takes a few weeks to "kick in."

Aspiration is a special formula for depression. It is designed to treat stagnant Qi and Blood, Dampness, and food and Phlegm entanglement. Many of the individual ingredients in this formula have anti-depressant actions. Aspiration has a warming and drying effect, therefore it should not be used with Heat signs.

Case Studies
Case 1
A patient with Bipolar syndrome (manic-depression) who had been off and on lithium for the past ten years, was given Aspiration by her practitioner. The patient reported that Aspiration taken at twelve tablets per day produced outstanding results. She found that her depression was not as severe when she stopped taking lithium. Many patients do not like taking lithium, because it reduces depression but also reduces the "high" or heightened mood elevation.

Case 2
A practitioner had a patient with insomnia and recommended Schizandra Dreams. The patient had good results with the formula, but after a week began to get leg cramps. The practitioner hypothesized that Schizandra Dreams, which contains calcium in the form of dragonbone and oystershell, upset the calcium/magnesium balance and therefore recommended a calcium-magnesium supplement; the leg cramps stopped.

Occasionally patients say that Schizandra Dreams does not work, which is usually due to not taking a large enough dose (some patients need five tablets before bed), or because patients take the formula too close to bedtime. It should be taken an hour before bedtime to give it time to calm the mind. Deeper-acting formulas such as Shen-Gem, Calm Spirit or Ease Plus may be necessary to get at the root of the insomnia.

Case 3
A female patient on antidepressant medication had loose stools, a history of endometriosis, a very pale complexion, deficient pulse, and a dry dark purple tongue. She took birth control pills, which can cause

Blood stagnation. The patient was put on Clearing for Yin tonification, loose stools, and Blood stagnation; and Woman's Balance for Liver Qi stagnation, depression, Heat signs (cold extremities, frequent thirst). I told this patient to take Clearing, two to three tablets TID, with one tablet of Woman's Balance, only every other day, since I was concerned that we might get a "Bupluerum reaction." In that reaction, Bupleurum helps to release the Liver's stored emotional anger all at one time.

The patient's tongue was better after three weeks and she had gone off the antidepressant medication (under medical supervision), but she was still feeling depressed. She reported fewer loose stools, but still some digestive problems. She had remarked earlier that salads and raw vegetables upset her stomach. I suggested cooked foods only and Quiet Digestion as needed. I had her start taking Aspiration every other day, three tablets TID, with Clearing and Woman's Balance dosage as before on alternate days.

After a few weeks the patient said that at first Aspiration really helped to bring up her energy and mood in a similar fashion to the antidepressants. However, after taking it for some time she felt it upset her digestion. I told her to take Clearing as before, and try taking in addition two tablets of Woman's Balance TID, and alternate Aspiration and Clearing on alternate days. She is doing much better and wondered if her menstrual period had thrown off her digestion and if it wasn't the Aspiration after all. The patient also needed to take Quiet Digestion from time to time. After six months she reported Aspiration had greatly helped her depression, and she found when she occasionally felt depressed she took Aspiration for a day, and her depression was lifted.

Analysis: This patient had a lot of Heat and stagnation, and cold extremities due to Liver stagnation. Aspiration may have been too drying and or tonifying (Damiana is a Kidney tonic) and so I suggested adding Women's Balance. I also told her to exercise more. I wasn't as concerned about the possible Bupluerum reaction after she had been taking it every other day for a few weeks. Generally patients get a Bupluerum effect if they have a lot of suppressed anger and then take a large dose every day.

Case 4

A patient with insomnia, migraines, anxiety and depression wondered whether Schizandra Dreams, Ease Plus and Calm Spirit could be taken together. The patient was on several medications for anxiety, depression, and insomnia.

Generally it is important to know whether or not the patient has constipation or loose stools. Calm Spirit is designed to be quickly effective. Often with these kinds of medications there is Heat and stagnation. Calm Spirit is designed to calm the Heart, however there is usually simultaneous Liver Qi stagnation. If the patient tends towards constipation, Calm Spirit and Ease Plus is a good choice. If the patient has loose stools, the Ease 2 will be a good counterbalance to Calm Spirit.

Schizandra Dreams can be taken in addition, five tablets an hour before bedtime. Shen-Gem is an excellent follow-up formula after two or three months as it nourishes the Heart Blood and tonifies the Spleen. Both Ease 2 and Ease Plus have herbs to protect the Stomach; nevertheless the patient will usually have a weak Spleen once all the excess symptoms are under control.

Case 5

A forty year-old woman with a slow pulse, normal tongue, and cold hands and feet, was suffering from depression due to the fact that her husband died, and was put on Aspiration. Since she was a sensitive patient she was told to take two tablets TID for the first week, and then three TID after that.

After four weeks she reported that she felt like "a new woman". It was springtime and she reported that she got a dry cough one hour after taking the Aspiration. I suggested that she cut down Aspiration slightly and see if the dry cough went away. I also suggested taking the herbs with an extra glass of water. If this did not help, or if the depression started creeping back, I suggested adding one or two tablets of Calm Spirit with the Aspiration, as this contains moistening herbs.

When a patient has particularly good results with a formula I try to modify it by taking it along with another formula, as opposed to selecting a different formula.

Case 6: Prozac Withdrawal

A thirty-four year-old woman on 80 mg of prozac per day (four times the normal dosage) saw a colleague who is a medical doctor. The woman was put on Aspiration and her dosage of Prozac was slowly withdrawn. Two months later she was taking nine tablets a day of Aspiration, was off Prozac, and "felt better than she ever did on Prozac."

Six months later, she took Aspiration only occasionally for a few days when she got depressed, and she was able to get relief for her depression.

Chronic Sweating and Night Sweats

Western Medicine

Night sweats can be the sign of cancer such as Hodgkin's disease, leukemia, and lymphomas; therefore medical diagnosis is extremely important. Sweating may accompany chest discomfort, signalling a heart attack, and is also found with hyperthyroidism, anxiety disorders, hypoglycemia, menopause, and pneumonia.

TCM

The most common form of sweating is associated with Yin deficiency. In this case it is called "five palm sweat" and is found on the palms, soles, and chest. If the whole body sweats, there is deficiency of Lung Qi; if there is sweat only on the head, it is due to Heat in the Stomach or Damp Heat. Daytime sweating is due to Yang deficiency and night sweats are usually due to Yin deficiency, although they can be due to Damp Heat. Damp Heat sweat tends to be yellow. Oily sweat suggests Yang deficiency.

Chinese Herbal Therapy

The most commonly seen patterns in American patients are Yin deficiency, Excess Heat, or Damp Heat. With Yin deficiency, I have successfully combined Nine Flavor Tea, which is suitable for long-term use, with Calm Spirit, which tonifies Heart Yin and relaxes the patient. Yin deficiency frequently affects a highly stressed individual who is "burning the candle at both ends." Night sweats due to Yin deficiency may also appear in patients taking pharmaceutical medications. In this presentation the tongue is red, the pulse is rapid, and the throat is dry at night. To get a stronger effect and to reduce empty fire, Coptis Purge Fire or Temper Fire (Zhi Bai Di Huang Wan) may be added until the fire is contained, at which point Nine Flavor Tea can be used for several months. If there is a weak digestive system, add Quiet Digestion or use Fertile Garden instead. Dryness can accompany sweating and is characterized by dry skin, lips, throat, and mouth, dry stools, and scanty urination.

If sweating is due to an Exterior invasion, use Isatis Gold. With Damp Heat use Phellostatin. With menopausal sweating use Two Immortals (see Menopause).

Case Studies
Case 1
A seventy-two year-old physician on high blood pressure medication, with blotchy red skin and night sweats so bad he had to get up once a night to change his pajamas, came for therapy. I recommended Calm Spirit, advising him to take three tablets TID between meals, and Nine Flavor Tea which I also suggested at three tablets TID. He also had prostate inflammation and had received three operations and was scheduled for a fourth, and had started to take Saw Palmetto berries tincture. I suggested that after two months he discontinue taking Calm Spirit and substitute Essence Chamber, and continue to take Saw Palmetto tincture.

Analysis: Night sweats are a classic symptom of Yin deficiency. The patient had other signs such as red blotchy skin and high blood pressure. He was put on two formulas because I wanted him to have improvement as soon as possible, since I surmised he would not take herbs for more than four to six weeks without results. It is often easier for patients to take eighteen pills of two formulas rather than of one formula.

I suggested he discontinue Calm Spirit and substitute Essence Chamber, since it would work on his other health problems, tonify the

> # Nine Flavor Tea
> ## Rehmannia 9 Formula
>
> Ingredients
>
> | English | *pinyin* |
> |---|---|
> | Rehmannia | Shu Di Huang and Sheng Di Huang |
> | Dioscorea | Shan Yao |
> | Poria | Fu Ling |
> | Cornus | Shan Zhu Yu |
> | Moutan | Mu Dan Pi |
> | Alisma | Ze Xie |
> | Dendrobium | Shi Hu |
> | Scrophularia | Xuan Shen |
> | Ophiopogon | Mai Men Dong |
>
> (see also: Calm Spirit, Coptis Purge Fire, Temper Fire, Isatis Cooling, Phellostatin, Two Immortals)

Yang, and serve as an adjunct to the tincture. Tinctures often do not have sufficient potency for this condition, according to some naturo-pathic researchers.

After two days the physician noted slight improvement, and after six weeks the night sweats were considerably reduced.

Case 2

A forty-eight year-old woman came in complaining of having burning feet for the past three years. She said she had been through all sorts of tests, and medical doctors said there was nothing much that could be done about her condition. She also complained of stress, and seemed angry and skeptical that she would get any benefit from the herbs. Her tongue was red without coating and her pulse was rapid.

I suggested a combination of Calm Spirit and Nine Flavor Tea. The dosage was two tablets of each TID. I included Calm Spirit because I suspected that if she didn't get quick relief she was going to give up on herbs. She came in four weeks later and reported that her feet no longer burned although sometimes they felt hot. She also complained of occa-sional stress headaches. At this point I kept her on Nine Flavor Tea, and decided to put her on Ease Plus, since I believed the source of the head-aches was rising Liver Yang.

Ulcers

Western Medicine

Ulcers of the stomach are called gastric ulcers; ulcers can also occur in the duodenum and colon. Ulcers are aggravated by stress. Aspirin, steroids, non-steroidal anti-inflammatory drugs and Vitamin C deficiency may contribute to stomach ulcers. Smokers frequently have ulcers.

TCM

Ulcers usually accompany Liver-invades-the-Spleen/Stomach. There can also be Blood stagnation, Qi stagnation, Stomach Yin deficiency and Liver Qi stagnation.

Chinese Herbal Therapy

(See also the appendix: Chinese Herbal Treatment of Chronic Digestive Disorders.)

If there is fullness, abdominal distension, pain in the upper abdomen, acid regurgitation, irritability, wiry pulse, and thin white tongue coating, Stomach Tabs is an excellent formula. If there is a burning sensation that does not get better with eating, and if the patient is thirsty, likes cold beverages, has a dry mouth with bitter taste, dark urine,

Stomach Tabs
Magnolia & Ginger Combination

Ingredients

English	pinyin
Magnolia bark	Hou Pu
Citrus	Chen Pi
Pinellia	Ban Xia
Red Atractylodes	Cang Zhu
Ginger	Gan Jiang
Licorice	Gan Cao
Bupleurum	Chai Hu
Oryza	Gu Ya

(see also: Clearing, Heavenly Water, Isatis Cooling, Flavonex, Six Gentlemen, Ease 2, Quiet Digestion)

red and greasy tongue with yellow coating, and a wiry rapid pulse, the Clearing formula may be used to treat Stomach Yin deficiency. Heavenly Water may be used simultaneously to relieve Liver Qi stagnation. If the pain is severe, as if being jabbed by an umbrella, or if there is intense burning, Isatis Cooling is usually very effective. This can be combined with Flavonex, a formula that has anti-inflammatory herbs and also promotes blood circulation. With Cold signs the Six Gentlemen with saussarea and cardamom is indicated. With loose stools use the Ease 2 formula.

Case Study

A patient had signs of Stomach Fire, with burning in the epigastrium, constant thirst, and red tongue. She had been in an auto accident six months earlier, which was why she came for acupuncture treatments. I suggested a combination of Isatis Cooling and Flavonex. The latter activates blood circulation and relieves inflammation. In this case, tinctures or warming Blood-activating formulas were not appropriate, because they would upset the Stomach Fire.

After taking two tablets of Isatis Cooling and two Flavonex TID, with weekly acupuncture, the patient showed an improvement in all symptoms.

Urinary Tract Infection, Urethritis, Cystitis

Western Medicine

Bladder infections are rarer in men than in woman, but may be more serious in men. In women, urinary tract infection (UTI) is usually caused by *Escherichia coli*, a bacteria found in the colon. Chlamydia may also cause bladder problems. Cranberry juice acidifies the urine, inhibiting bacterial growth. Hot baths help relieve pain associated with cystitis. One cup of vinegar may be added once per day to a bath. Legs and knees must be positioned so that water can enter the urethra.

TCM

Cystitis and urethritis may accompany Damp Heat in the Lower Burner.

Chinese Herbal Therapy

Akebia Moist Heat has been very effective in the treatment of cystitis. It is often helpful to increase the dosage for the first few days to three tablets every three to four hours, and then three tablets TID.

Clearing is formulated specifically for chronic bladder infections. Use it as a follow-up after using the Akebia Moist Heat for two bottles or when the symptoms have gone, whichever is longer. If a woman has frequent infections, Clearing should be used for a minimum of three to six months.

Case Studies

Case 1

A lawyer in her mid-thirties who had been on several courses of antibiotics for frequent urinary tract infections came in for herbs. She was given two bottles of Akebia Moist Heat and told to take three tablets TID. As a follow-up she took with her two bottles of Clearing. Although she was supposed to continue taking Clearing, she decided not to come back in, and has not had a UTI in more than one year. She felt that herbs were very successful.

Analysis: Akebia Moist Heat treats the acute stage of UTI, whereas Clearing is a treatment for chronic UTI. Akebia Moist Heat contains Damp Heat-resolving herbs; Clearing clears Heat, but also tonifies the Spleen and Blood.

Akebia Moist Heat

Ingredients

English	pinyin
Akebia	Mu Tong
Tetrapanax	Tong Cao
Juncus	Deng Xin Cao
Benincassa	Dong Gua Zi
Tricosanthes root	Tian Hua Fen
Dianthus	Qu Mai
Coix	Yi Yi Ren
Alisma	Ze Xie
Magnesium salts	Hua Shi
Aristolochia	Ma Dou Ling
Polyporus	Zhu Ling
Sophora	Ku Shen
Smilax	Tu Fu Ling
Platycodon	Jie Geng
Aster	Zi Wan
Nutgall	Mo Shi Zi
Cuttlebone	Hai Piao Xiao
Mume	Wu Mei

(see also: Clearing)

Case 2

A twenty-five year-old woman got results within a few days taking Akebia Moist Heat for cystitis. She was extremely impressed.

Case 3

A forty-six year-old woman with deficiency of Kidney Yin and Yang and a long history of bladder problems reported that she was having bladder spasms and frequent urination. She was given Astra Essence to tonify Kidney Yin and Yang and also because it is astringent. Crampbark Plus was also recommended as an antispasmodic. I recommended two tablets of Astra Essence and two Crampbark Plus TID. I suggested she take an additional three tablets of Crampbark Plus if her spasms continued, but I cautioned her against taking more than nine tablets per day of the Crampbark Plus, as any more might upset her dry Lung. Like many patients, she appeared to have Heat in the Lung but Coldness in the Lower Burner. The Heat and dryness were not severe, which was why I felt she didn't need a more moistening formula.

After one week she reported a dramatic reduction in bladder spasms. Treatment will continue using the two formulas.

Uterine Fibroids

Western Medicine

Uterine fibroids rarely cause symptoms before the age of thirty. These benign tumors can interfere with the bladder, causing urinary frequency and dysuria. They may also grow around the endometrium causing menorrhagia and dysmenorrhea; they may also press on the rectum causing tenesmus. A gynecological exam is important to make sure the fibroid tumors are not cancerous. If there is an unusually rapid growth of tumors, they must be removed.

TCM

Fibroids can be caused by stagnation of Qi or Blood, or by Phlegm accumulation.

Chinese Herbal Therapy

Bupleurum Entangled Qi has been successfully used as it contains several ingredients such as Cyperus (Xiang Fu), that resolve lumps and swellings. This formula will be more effective if combined with Crampbark Plus for Cold signs, or with Unlocking for Heat signs, as the latter two formulas are specifically directed to the uterus. The recommended dosage is two tablets of each formula TID or QID.

Unlocking
Damp Heat Dysmenorrhea Tablets

Ingredients

English	pinyin
Patrinia	Bai Jiang Cao
St. John's Wort	Yuan Bao Cao
Sargentodoxa	Da Xue Teng
Cyathula	Chuan Niu Xi
Melia	Chuan Lian Zi
Moutan	Mu Dan Pi
Red Peony	Chi Shao
Dioscorea	Shan Yao
Cuscuta	Tu Su Zi
Poria	Fu Ling
Fennel	Xiao Hui Xiang

(see also: Bupleurum Entangled Qi, Crampbark Plus)

Notes

Herbal therapy will be more successful when combined with a low-fat diet that minimizes alcohol and coffee.

Case Study

A colleague reported that her patient had a uterine fibroid the size of a softball. After receiving acupuncture, taking Bupleurum Entangled Qi, and following the above mentioned dietary modifications, the patient's fibroid was the size of a pea after several months.

Appendix A
Chinese Herbal Treatment of Chronic Digestive Disorders

Digestive disorders are extremely common in the United States. Chronic flatulence, tiredness after eating, heartburn, fullness of the stomach, abdominal bloating, sharp stabbing abdominal pain, diarrhea, and constipation — all common signs of chronic digestive disorders — are all common in the population.

Many Americans consume antacids in large quantities but do not even consider themselves to be suffering from a digestive disorder. The American dietary habits of eating on the run, consuming cold and raw foods, drinking iced beverages, and eating large quantities of dairy products, sweets, fried foods, and alcohol, are perhaps the greatest contributing factors to digestive disorders.

Proper digestion is necessary for good health. Undigested or incompletely digested food molecules that are absorbed into the system can lead to various diseases and the development of food allergies. Conditions of the small intestine often cause malabsorption syndromes. This article discusses the traditional Chinese medicine (TCM) syndromes and treatment of the following biomedical diseases: ulcerative colitis, Crohn's disease, peptic ulcers, and irritable bowel syndrome.

Symptoms and Syndrome Patterns

TCM treatment of diseases is based on the correct differentiation of syndrome patterns. Thus, while the Western diagnosis of some conditions may differ, the TCM pattern may be the same. For example, Crohn's disease and ulcerative colitis are different according to biomedicine but may have the same underlying TCM pattern. Crohn's disease is characterized by an inflammatory reaction throughout the entire bowel wall; the condition is also known as regional ileitis. The disease can last for many years with exacerbations and remissions of symptoms that include diarrhea, abdominal pain, anemia, weight loss, fistula formation, and eventual intestinal obstruction. Stools are soft and grayish or brownish, with abundant fecal particles. Any part of the gastrointestinal tract may be involved, but the ileum is the most common site. Current Western treatment is usually long-term antibiotic or steroid therapy.

Ulcerative colitis is characterized by passage of watery stools with mucus and pus. Accompanying symptoms may include abdominal pain, tenderness or colic, as well as intermittent or irregular fever. Serious cases may present hemorrhaging and perforation.

Both Crohn's disease and ulcerative colitis are considered inflammatory bowel diseases (IBD). Men between fifteen and thirty-five years of age are most commonly affected. In 15-40% of cases, multiple members of a family are sufferers of Crohn's disease or ulcerative colitis. Although immune dysfunction is common in IBD, it is unclear if it is the cause or the result of IBD. The actual cause of IBD is unknown. A virus or bacteria may be at fault, or a breakdown of the body's immune system, or a combination of the two. IBD is not caused by emotional stress, although flare-ups may occur during such times.

Irritable bowel syndrome (IBS) is also quite common in the U.S. IBS is not associated with pathologic changes in the intestine, or with inflammation. It is widely believed that emotional fluctuations play a strong role in causing IBS. Also known as spastic colon or nervous indigestion, IBS symptoms include abdominal pain and distention with relief after bowel movement; constipation, diarrhea, excess mucus production in the colon, and indigestion.

A peptic ulcer, which occurs in the upper gastrointestinal tract, is a circumscribed ulceration of the mucous membrane penetrating through the muscularis mucosa. The most common type of peptic ulcer, a duodenal ulcer, is found in the first few centimeters of the duodenum. Another common form occurs along the lesser curvature of the stomach and is known as a gastric ulcer. The typical pattern of pain in patients with duodenal ulcers is: It is absent upon wakening in the morning, but appears in mid-morning; it is relieved by food, but recurs two to three hours after a meal; pain that awakens the patient at 1 or 2 AM is common. The symptoms of gastric ulcer often do not follow the duodenal ulcer pattern, and eating may cause rather than relieve the pain. Certain drugs, especially aspirin, other nonsteroidal anti-inflammatory drugs, and possibly corticosteroids, predispose to the formation of upper gastrointestinal ulcers that tend to heal when the drug is discontinued.

In diagnosing chronic digestive disorders, parasitic infections and food allergies must be ruled out. Gastroenterologists generally recommend a low-fiber diet, although good nutrition is very important, especially for IBD sufferers, since anemia is quite common. Successful treatment of chronic digestive disorders necessitates first treating any parasitic and/or candida infections that may be present.

According to TCM, the spirit in which food is eaten during meals is very important. Concentration should be focused on eating. Worrying or thinking while eating may cause the body harm. Also, returning to work immediately after a meal or working while eating could compromise the digestive process.

Many Americans tend to be Qi deficient, which affects both our energy and our ability to convert foods into energy. Chemical medications as well as recreational drugs may induce Stomach Yin deficiency. The root of digestive disorders is usually Liver Qi invading the Spleen/Stomach. Stagnant Liver Qi disrupts the ability of the Spleen to transform food into energy. When stagnation of Liver Qi predominates, constipation with tiny dry stools is a common presentation; with Spleen deficiency, stools are loose. Other symptoms of Liver and Spleen/Stomach Qi stagnation include distention, fullness in the upper abdomen that is aggravated after meals or by emotional stress, frequent belching, pain relieved by bowel movements, nausea, regurgitation, and a thin white tongue coating.

Individuals who are in the habit of drinking cold beverages and eating ice cream and raw foods are particularly prone to a Cold Damp pattern. Their symptoms include pain that is relieved by pressure, distention and fullness of the stomach after meals, tiredness, cold limbs, pale tongue with white coating and a weak pulse.

A burning pain in the upper abdomen relieved by meals, thirst without the desire to drink much, irritability, red tongue with dry yellow coating, and a rapid pulse all point to Yin deficiency pattern.

In all chronic digestive disorders food stagnation is present. Chronic Dampness precludes complete digestion of food. Overeating, eating too quickly, or eating while emotionally upset can all lead to food stagnation. Symptoms include a sensation of fullness in the stomach, foul breath, sour regurgitation, belching, and insomnia, along with a thick yellow or white tongue coating.

Damp Heat in the Large Intestine is another common syndrome of chronic digestive disorders. Qi deficiency is also present along with abdominal pain, diarrhea, mucus and blood in the stools, smelly stools, heaviness in the body, fever, anal burning, and a red tongue with a sticky yellow coating. Individuals with this pattern are generally diagnosed as having candidiasis by holistic physicians whether or not tests indicate higher than normal candida counts. Many cases of candidiasis are iatrogenic because of the over-prescribing of antibiotics by Western physicians. When colonies of yeast are established in the mucous membranes, they can survive for years and even decades if the patient's diet is composed of high sugar, yeast, or fermented foods. Yeast can attach to the wall of the colon, small intestine, or any other part of the gastrointestinal tract, and release toxic by-products into the circulatory system. These by-products inhibit the function of T-suppressor cells. According to Seattle physician Ralph Golan, M.D. *(The New Medicine Guide,* Ballantine Books, 1994), a yeast-impaired immune system has less than normal tolerance for ordinarily safe levels of common chemicals such as gasoline and oil fumes, cleaning fluids, and pesticide residues found on supermarket produce. Dr. Golan also notes that an impaired immune system may produce antibodies to the body's own tissues resulting in autoimmune diseases. Other pharmaceuticals that may lead to candidiasis include cortisone, immunosuppressants, and birth control pills. Patients suffering Crohn's disease or colitis have a propensity for developing both candidiasis and Damp Heat in the Intestines. Thus, in addition to following a TCM diet, herbs in a well-balanced formula should be taken for extended periods. Severe cases of IBD involve Blood stasis, which is characterized by fixed stabbing pain, a tongue that is purple in the center, dark blood in the stools, and epigastric pain. Because inflammation is a major symptom of IBD, the standard medical treatment is long-term administration of steroids, antibiotics, or sulfa drugs. Surgery is now rare because steroids are almost immediately effective. However, TCM views the use of steroids as harmful to the Kidney. And from a Western medicine standpoint, steroids may cause gastrointestinal disorders and a myriad of other problems. Long-term antibiotic use may cause gastrointestinal complaints, fungal overgrowth, and allergic reactions. Sulfa drugs may also lead to gastrointestinal disturbances and allergic skin reactions.

Treatment

Chinese herbs that have an anti-inflammatory action are excellent not only in reducing inflammation, but also in attacking bacteria which may be the cause of flare-ups of IBD. Isatis leaf (Da Qing Ye) and root (Ban Lan Gen) are very effective as they are both antibiotic and antiviral, according to Chinese research. They are also Cool in nature, and thus are anti-inflammatory. In studies described by Bensky and Gamble in *Chinese Herbal Medicine: Materia Medica*, 300 patients were administered Isatis and their "fevers would usually disappear entirely within one day, and frequency of bowel movements usually returned to normal within five days" (p. 127). Smilax (Tu Fu Ling) is also an important herb which clears Damp Heat poison and treats ulcers. According to Michael Murray, N.D., in his *Healing Power of Herbs* (p. 215), Smilax is an endo-toxin binder. Endotoxins are cell wall constituents of bacteria that are absorbed in the gut. If the liver is in dysfunction, the endotoxins may seep into the bloodstream and activate the alternate complement system which plays a critical role in the inflammatory process.

Among Health Concerns' formulas, Phellostatin is perhaps the most suitable for treating IBD especially because of its antifungal properties, since many IBD patients are also afflicted by candidiasis. The main ingredient is Phellodendron (Huang Bai) which treats diarrhea and eliminates Heat and Dampness. The remaining herbs in the formula tonify the Qi, clear Heat and Dampness, and are anti-inflammatory and antifungal. Phellostatin may be combined with Quiet Digestion. The primary ingredient in the latter formula is Shen Qu which is composed of fermented herbs that are rich in enzymatic activity. For severe cases of gas and bloating, Quiet Digestion may be taken every two hours until the gas subsides. The formula is designed to break down rapidly in the gut for immediate relief. It should be started slowly, one tablet TID, and then gradually increased to three tablets TID after two to three weeks. Quiet Digestion is taken just before meals in order to help the assimilation of food. It may also be taken after meals when gas-inducing foods are consumed, usually two tablets until the symptoms are alleviated. We recommend combining Quiet Digestion with other formulas when treating chronic digestive disorders, since food stagnation is so common among these cases.

For chronic digestive disorders that are accompanied by pain and inflammation, Isatis Cooling is appropriate. In addition to Isatis extract (Da Qing Ye and Ban Lan Gen), its other ingredients tonify the Spleen, promote blood circulation, clear Dampness and Heat, and are anti-inflammatory, antifungal, and antibacterial. Under proper medical supervision Isatis Cooling may be tried as steroids are slowly withdrawn. Underlying the Heat and inflammation is deficiency; thus after a course of Phellostatin or Isatis Cooling, Six Gentlemen may be used to tonify the Spleen (especially in a Cold pattern), or Astra Essence, a balanced formula with Kidney Yin, Yang, and Blood tonics.

Stomach Tabs have proven to be an effective remedy in the treatment of IBS and peptic ulcers. Based on Ping Wei San (Relieve the Stomach Powder), this formula is modified with Bupleurum since many individuals with chronic digestive disorders tend to repress their emotions; it is also included for its anti-inflammatory effect. The other herbs in the formula stimulate digestive enzymes, remove Phlegm, treat gas, and remove food stagnation.

For Stomach Yin deficiency pattern, Clearing should be used instead because it does not contain Rehmannia (Shu Di Huang) which some patients cannot tolerate; it can be cloying and may aggravate the symptoms of chronic digestive disorder.

The above formulas are very effective in treating the complex syndrome patterns that are presented in patients with IBD, IBS, and ulcers. I have been using prepared formulas with much success. They are often better-tolerated than teas. Sufferers of chronic digestive disorders generally have malabsorption problems, thus herbal teas may not be suitable, because they are absorbed too quickly to be effective in these patients. Interestingly, persons with digestive conditions are unusually sensitive, in particular to bitter tastes, so that again, herbal teas may not be well tolerated. Perhaps these individuals would do well to consume more bitter substances as prescribed in the European tradition which encourages taking herbal "bitters" for indigestion. Herbal teas, however, should not be eliminated completely from the therapeutic regimen. I generally advise clients to drink at least three cups of hot peppermint tea daily, because this herb relieves stomach and bowel spasms and alleviates nausea. On occasion I have also administered simple, pleasant-tasting herbal decoctions with herbal tablets in order to tonify the Qi and Blood. Therefore, by using teas and tablets, patients can consume more herbs; inexperienced practitioners often do not use high enough dosages. Since conventional medical treatment for chronic digestive disorders is not very promising, there is a great opportunity for Chinese medicine to help this large group of patients. As practitioners we should encourage ourselves to be more outspoken about the power of alternative medicines in healing diseases that are often un-healable in Western medicine.

Treatment of specific conditions

Heartburn

The most common malady among Americans is indigestion, which may include stomach pain, nausea, vomiting, gas, belching, or heartburn. Ten percent of Americans suffer heartburn daily. Common symptoms are burning pain behind the breast bone and acid regurgitation.

Cigarette smoking, tomato products, chocolate, coffee, citrus fruits and juices, and of course fried or fatty foods, can all cause heartburn, as can individual sensitivities. Relief for most people comes from standing upright or from taking antacids. The latter, if used for a long time, may lead to diarrhea, altered calcium metabolism (calcium-containing products such as Tums actually increase stomach acid secretion), and magnesium retention. It should be mentioned that heartburn is not caused by hiatal hernia, in which the stomach protrudes through an opening in the diaphragm at the junction of the esophagus and stomach.

For acid regurgitation with Heat signs, the classic Chinese formula is Left Metal Pill (Zuo Jin Wan). The chief herb, Coptis (Huang Lian), drains Liver Fire and clears Heat from the Stomach. The assistant herb, Evodia (Wu Zhu Yu), disperses Liver constraint and brings Stomach Qi downward. A modification of this formula, known as Coptis and Evodia Formula, is available from Seven Forests. According to Bensky and Barolet in *Chinese Herbal Medicine: Formulas & Strategies*, Left Metal Pill may also be used in treating hernial disorders with a similar presentation (p. 99). The modification includes Peony (Bai Shao) which disperses constrained Liver Qi.

A formula that I have used successfully to treat chronic heartburn is Ease Plus, which is based on Bupleurum Plus Dragon Bone and Oyster Shell Decoction (Chai Hu Jia Long Gu Mu Li Tang). A patient with heartburn who was diagnosed as having chronic esophagitis and who had symptoms of Liver overacting on the Spleen, along with Spleen Qi deficiency symptoms such as fatigue, responded quite favorably to Ease Plus. The calcium-containing herbs of Dragonbone (Long Gu) and Oystershell (Mu Li) absorb acidity and calm the Spirit, while Ginseng (Ren Shen) tonifies the Spleen. For simple occasional heartburn, another formula, Quiet Digestion, is effective.

Acid regurgitation may also be brought on by a Cold Spleen, usually the result of injury from cold foods. Six Gentlemen may be used in this case to harmonize the function of the Stomach and Spleen, and to promote the flow of Qi.

Constipation

Treating constipation is big business in the U.S. Patients as well as practitioners should understand that the normal frequency of bowel movements in healthy individuals ranges greatly. Constipation is a symptom that can signal a more serious disease, though it is frequently related to travel, low- fiber diet, medications, or repeatedly ignoring the urge to defecate.

Chronic constipation may be a symptom of irritable bowel syndrome (IBS), parasitic infection, hormonal imbalance, hemorrhoids, disease affecting the body tissues, nerve damage, and laxative abuse. The latter includes natural laxatives and colon cleansers found over-the-counter.

In Chinese medicine, constipation commonly suggests Heat, though in the elderly or postpartum women it may be due to deficiency of Blood. It may also be associated with extreme internal Cold and Yang deficiency.

A simple and effective formula is Gentle Senna, developed by Dr. Fung Fung on the basis of his 60 years' experience with Chinese herbs. This formula moistens the intestines and unblocks the bowels.

Calm Spirit, a formula designed to treat stress-related emotions, contains Biota (Bai Zi Ren), Tang-kuei (Dang Gui), and Ophiopogon (Mai Men Dong), to moisten the intestines. The remaining herbs, in addition to calming the Spirit, nourish the Blood and Yin. For Type A personalities who suffer from insomnia, restlessness, and constipation, I suggest using Ease Plus in addition to Calm Spirit. For constipation due to Blood deficiency, Eight Treasures may be used, and for Cold and Yang deficiency, the formulas Backbone or Rehmannia 8. Individuals on laxatives or colon cleansers should be weaned slowly from these remedies even while taking Chinese herbs that help moisten the intestines.

Diarrhea

Another Large Intestine problem is diarrhea, which can be caused by either Cold or by Damp Heat. For Spleen Qi deficiency exhibiting Cold symptoms, the tongue coating is white and the pulse is slow; for Damp Heat, the tongue coating is yellow and the pulse rapid. Other manifestations include tiredness of the four limbs in Spleen Qi deficiency, as contrasted by heaviness of the limbs in Damp Heat conditions; fever may be present in Damp Heat, but not in cases of Spleen Qi deficiency.

An excellent Spleen Qi tonic is Astra 8. This formula contains Schizandra (Wu Wei Zi) which stops diarrhea. Astra 8 may be combined with a Kidney Yang tonic for best results, since many individuals with Spleen Qi deficiency also have Kidney Yang deficiency. Kidney Yang tonics such as Rehmannia 8 or Backbone are helpful in such cases. Because these formulas are warming in nature, they are contraindicated with signs of Heat such as thirst, red tongue, rapid pulse, dark, scanty, or painful urination, insomnia, red eyes, or bleeding due to Heat in the Blood.

For diarrhea due to chronic Damp Heat, the formula Phellostatin is quite effective. This remedy helps rid the body of candida which may be present in individuals presenting with Damp Heat. Chronic Damp Heat conditions are common among Americans because of our fast-paced lifestyle and a diet that includes alcohol, caffeinated beverages, fast foods, sweets, dairy products, and the like. Therapeutic and recreational drugs also contribute to the problem. Phellostatin can be taken with Quiet Digestion, and started at a reduced dosage. One last word about Damp Heat: persons with chronic Damp Heat often have concomitant Spleen Qi deficiency because Dampness absorbs the body's energy which is in part devoted to nourishment.

Diarrhea that arises from traveling, food poisoning, or stomach flu is effectively countered with Quiet Digestion. The usual dosage is one or two tablets every two hours. Although enzyme formulas containing pancreatin are effective short-term, they are not recommended for prolonged use since they interfere with the body's own production of pancreatin.

Gallstones

More than twenty-five million Americans suffer from gallstones. Women between the ages of 20 and 60 are three times more likely to develop gallstones as are men. Women who are overweight, have been pregnant, or who have used oral menopausal estrogen therapy are at greater risk of developing gallstones. Gallstones can also develop in women soon after they lose weight. Symptoms of gallstones include intense abdominal pain, bloating, gas, nausea, and discomfort following the consumption of fatty foods. Currently, oral ursodiol is used to dissolve stones. However, there is a seventy percent recurrence rate. Cholecystectomy, the surgical removal of the gallbladder, is one of the most common surgical procedures. This should be a last resort, since surgery weakens the body and puts the patient at risk for developing secondary infections associated with hospital visits. Finally, removal of the gallbladder may have energetic consequences that we do not yet fully understand.

An empirical formula, GB-6, is used in China to prevent and eliminate gallstones, and to treat the discomfort associated with gallbladder inflammation. In Chinese clinics, after an acute attack which is treated with decoctions, GB-6 is administered as a follow-up therapy for three months. American practitioners have given this formula as a follow-up to ursodiol and surgery, since surgery may not relieve the symptoms of pain, gas, bloating, nausea, and accumulated Damp Heat.

It should be noted that the "liver flush" remedy of lemon and olive oil is actually counterproductive. The main constituent of olive oil, oleic acid, has been found experimentally to increase the risk of developing gallstones. Furthermore, consuming large quantities of oil constricts the gallbladder, thus increasing the chances of a gallstone blocking the bile duct *(Encyclopedia of Natural Medicine*, p. 325).

Diverticulosis

Diverticula are small, saccular, mucosal herniations through the muscular wall of the colon. They occur anywhere in the colon, but most often in the sigmoid. Inflammation of one or more diverticula is known as diverticulitis. Symptoms of inflammation include fever, abdominal pain, and an elevated white blood cell count. Treatment usually involves bed rest, pain relievers, antibiotics, and intravenous fluids. Surgery may be required if an abscess, fistula, or perforation develops.

Isatis Cooling is a formula that I have used successfully to treat patients with Crohn's disease, colitis, or painful IBS. It can also be used effectively in conjunction with biomedical therapy for diverticulitis. The presenting syndrome pattern is that of Blood stagnation which is characterized by constant, fixed, stabbing pain, bruises or dark blotches of the skin, and a purple tongue. For cases that also present with Qi stagnation, Aquilaria 22 can be included in the therapeutic regimen. Common symptoms of Qi stagnation include pain that is non-fixed, distention, feeling of fullness, depression, mood swings, and frequent sighing. Aquilaria 22 can also help alleviate constipation.

If chronic loose stools are associated with diverticulitis, a more conservative formula is Six Gentlemen, which contains Citrus (Chen Pi) and Saussurea (Mu Xiang) to relieve Qi stagnation. To assist digestion, another formula, Quiet Digestion, can be used before and after each meal along with Aquilaria 22 or Six Gentlemen. Longer-term therapy can involve Six Gentlemen and Astra Essence, when Kidney deficiency is present. A stronger Kidney tonic such as Rehmannia 8 or Backbone may be used when there is obvious Kidney Yang deficiency.

Gluten Intolerance

This condition is also known as celiac disease. It is a malabsorption syndrome brought on by ingesting gluten-containing foods, primarily wheat and rye, and to a lesser degree barley and oat products. Potato and rice products must be substituted. Furthermore, gluten is so widely used that patients must be exceedingly wary of what they eat. Even herbal formulas that contain gluten both as active or inert ingredients must be avoided, including Chinese patent medicines that have malt (Mai Ya). Symptoms of gluten intolerance include abdominal distention, flatulence, weight loss, fatigue, anemia, difficulty in breathing, and stools that are bulky, frothy, fatty, and malodorous. Other symptoms of malabsorption and malnutrition may be present. One formula that addresses many of the acute digestive symptoms is Stomach Tabs, which is tolerated quite well.

Concluding Remarks

Individuals who are not responding to herbal therapy should undergo further tests for parasite infection; here I would like to add gluten intolerance as another consideration for additional testing.

A final area where Chinese herbs have a major impact is post-surgical recovery. Many individuals suffer food stagnation as well as general Qi and Blood deficiency after surgery. An excellent formula for these cases is Quiet Digestion, which addresses food stagnation. It can be combined with Six Gentlemen and Eight Treasures which tonify Qi and Blood and eliminate Dampness.

In my estimation, the etiology of many chronic digestive disorders is congenital Kidney Yang deficiency, which leads to Spleen Qi deficiency, and then to Dampness. Poor dietary and lifestyle habits induce the accumulation of Dampness which transforms into Damp Heat. Successful treatment of digestive disorders warrants the correct analysis and application of the correct formula for the presenting syndrome pattern.

Appendix B
Treating CFIDS in the Clinic

Most people with chronic fatigue immune deficiency syndrome (CFIDS), respond favorably to treatment with Chinese herbs. Those with mild conditions may report marked improvement within a week or two of starting on herbs, but many persons will be on herbs for several months before their symptoms take a significant turn for the better.

Practitioners must keep in mind that each case should be approached individually. The common symptoms of CFIDS are extreme fatigue, sleep disturbance, difficulty concentrating, memory loss, anxiety, depression, irritability, fever, sore throat, swollen lymph nodes, digestive disorders, sensitivity to heat and light, headaches, spasms, aching muscles and joints, recurrent infections (especially of the respiratory tract), and loss of appetite. Many persons also suffer from candidiasis or parasitosis.

To address the chronic fatigue in these patients, I suggest the use of Power Mushrooms or other mushroom extracts; most CFIDS patients feel more energetic after taking these formulas. Medicinal mushrooms may have anti-viral effects as well. For some Yin-deficient individuals, the mushroom formulas may be too warming, therefore these patients should be monitored closely for Heat signs.

Many CFIDS sufferers have problems with digestion, often due to Dampness and food stagnation. Thus, before starting them on other formulas, a two-week regimen of Quiet Digestion will usually help them handle the other herbs that are to come. Ordinarily, Quiet Digestion is taken between meals, but if the condition is more serious, the dosage should be increased to one tablet before and after meals. This initial step with Quiet Digestion can be bypassed if the digestive symptoms are mild or absent altogether.

Yeast infections such a vaginal candidiasis or oral thrush should also be treated. Even though there may be no obvious symptoms, if the patient has been on long-term antibiotics or oral contraceptives, the possibility that candida is present is high. Phellostatin is quite effective for candidiasis; herbs in this formula have been shown through laboratory studies to possess anti-candida properties. In Chinese medicine, the pattern of candidiasis fits that of Damp Heat lodged in the Spleen/Stomach and Intestines. This may be the causative factor of the aching muscles and joints experienced by CFIDS sufferers. Other symptoms of Damp

Heat in the Spleen/Stomach and Intestines are abdominal discomfort, diarrhea, mucus and blood in the stools, sweating, and thirst. Phellostatin is ordinarily taken for several months and can be combined with acidophilus, pharmaceuticals, and with other formulas such as Astra Isatis.

For viral infections, Astra Isatis has proved to be effective not only in treating chronic viremia, but also in resolving Kidney Yin and Yang deficiencies, since any type of chronic condition will affect the Kidney. Individuals with active viral symptoms, however, should be given Clear Heat, one to three tablets TID, since they usually present a pattern of Heat, and experience fever, a sensation of heat or burning in the muscles and joints of the extremities, a red tongue, and a rapid pulse. We have received reports that patients who have taken Clear Heat experience a dramatic reduction in joint and muscle pain when it is due to viral infection. It is suggested that Clear Heat be taken with Astra Isatis, which protects the Spleen/Stomach from the cooling herbs in Clear Heat. It should also be noted that even though some CFIDS patients do not exhibit outright signs of viral infection, it is advisable that they still be administered an anti-viral remedy. Following a severe viral infection, many persons will suffer extreme Yin deficiency. This is manifested by chronic sore throat, thirst, ulcers of the mouth, facial flush, afternoon fever, night sweats, and burning palms and soles. For these patients, Nine Flavors Tea, a modification of Liu Wei Di Huang Wan (Rehmannia Six), helps tonify the Yin and is the primary formula, although Astra Isatis may still be taken to eliminate residual viremia. Another important ingredient in Nine Flavor Tea is Scrophularia (Xuan Shen) which helps relieve lymph node swelling. Practitioners must be vigilant of CFIDS patients who have difficulty digesting Yin tonics, since these remedies can be cloying. If this is so, then Fertile Garden may be substituted.

If there are no signs of active viremia, Astra Isatis can be administered alone, or in combination with formulas that address specific symptoms. For example, mental depression with Cold signs is treated effectively with Aspiration; however, depression with Heat signs and anxiety, is better resolved with Calm Spirit. High levels of liver enzymes are also common in CFIDS patients, in which case Ecliptex may be administered. For PMS and menstrual cramps, Woman's Balance and Crampbark Plus may be used, respectively. For obvious Cold patterns, Astra Eight is effective since it tonifies the Spleen and Lung Qi.

For long-term therapy, Enhance, which was developed for HIV patients, can be alternated with Astra Isatis; it is generally beneficial to alternate formulas rather than use a single formula for a long time. Also, Enhance contains herbs that remove Blood stasis which often accompanies protracted illness.

Biomedical scientists are uncertain what virus or combination of viruses causes CFIDS, although some patients exhibit high levels of the Epstein-Barr virus. CFIDS is a complex condition for which there is no single remedy — overcoming it requires a multi-pronged approach. While herbal treatment is important, the patient's diet is just as significant. Practitioners should counsel their clients about a well-balanced diet that includes cooked foods, grains, fresh vegetables, and which minimizes sweets, and greasy or cold foods. Also, nutritional supplements (e.g., vitamins and otherwise) are generally warming in nature, and can lead to Yin deficiency and even Damp Heat. Thus, CFIDS sufferers should either avoid these products or use them only under the supervision of a knowledgeable practitioner or physician.

Patients should also be cautioned about rebound symptoms — the result of "over-doing it." That is, just as they are beginning to experience a return to health, they over-exert themselves, causing a relapse. Gentle exercise is the key. Finally, collaboration with a supportive MD is helpful, particularly for a diagnosis to rule out other conditions such as infectious and endocrine diseases, anemia and parasitosis.

Appendix C
Integrating Chinese Herbs and Western Medicine in the Treatment of HIV

For more than two thousand years, herbalists in China have pre-scribed herbs to build up the natural defenses of patients. Epidemics were common throughout Chinese history, and famous doctors such as Zhang Zhongjing used herbal formulas to treat individuals suffering from epidemic diseases.

Since 1949, the Chinese have applied a combination of traditional and Western medicines to treat immune disorders. The term *fu zheng* was coined to describe this type of therapeutic regimen: the use of herbs to enhance the natural host defense mechanism. In 1975, doctors in China organized an extensive fu zheng study to test the efficacy of tradi-tional formulas in pill form on cancer patients undergoing chemother-apy and radiation therapy. Almost one thousand patients were enrolled. The initial results found that patients who underwent the combined fu zheng and Western therapies tolerated treatment better and survived longer than those who underwent Western treatment alone. Ten-year fol-low-up studies have confirmed these findings. The most common herb used in the fu zheng formulas is Astragalus (Huang Qi).

Early U.S. Fu Zheng Studies

Based on the Chinese experience in treating immune-suppressed cancer patients, practitioners in the U.S. applied similar principles in treating HIV-infected patients. In 1986, the Immune Enhancement Proj-ect became the first study undertaken in this country. Twenty patients with AIDS-related complex (ARC) were administered Astra 8 and a mushroom formula comprised of Ganoderma (Ling Zhi, or Reishi) and Shiitake. Using a self-monitoring checklist, the participants evaluated the following symptoms prior to starting on the herbs, and at one month, two month, and three month intervals: fatigue, diarrhea, consti-pation, weight loss, nausea, gastrointestinal problems, leukoplakia, diffi-culties at night (including night sweats, frequent urination, insomnia, vivid dreaming), lymphadenopathy, sinus problems, oral fungus, skin problems, leg/knee weakness, tumors, herpes, neurological changes, emotional instability, and antibiotic use.

The twenty patients exhibited improvement in nearly all of the tabu-lated symptoms, with fatigue and lymphadenopathy showing the great-est changes. In all patients, diarrhea and night sweats were all but resolved, and of the eleven patients who were taking antibiotics at the beginning of the study, only one was doing so at the end of the three months. The practitioners who oversaw the Immune Enhancement Project were Lisa Hill, L.Ac., Jay Sordean, L.Ac., OMD, and Susan Black, L.Ac., R.N.

In 1989, a small study was conducted at Bastyr College of Natural Health Sciences in Seattle using Astra Isatis, vitamins and minerals, and other naturopathic approaches to treat AIDS patients. Subjects who completed the study experienced considerable improvement of their symptoms.

Since 1984, various treatment programs for HIV, hepatitis, and other viral diseases have been conducted at Quan Yin Healing Arts Center in San Francisco. Quan Yin has probably treated more HIV-infected patients with acupuncture and Chinese herbs than anywhere else in the world. In so doing, it has provided special training for the many American practitioners who treat HIV patients. Quan Yin's treatment philosophy is to enhance the immune system with Chinese herbs (fu zheng), and to clear Heat and Toxin using antiviral therapies.

Other attempts to monitor treatment results using Chinese herbs include a study done in 1987 at Quan Yin which used granulated herbs and involved twenty-nine patients. Then, in 1988, a formal investigation of herbal formulas was begun at Quan Yin and ultimately led to a formula called Composition A. As reported by Makima Hawkins, L.Ac., and colleagues, at the 1993 "HIV, AIDS, and Chinese Medicine" conference held in San Francisco, half of the symptoms monitored, including fatigue, night sweats, fever/chills, anxiety, depression, lymphadenopathy, and headache, showed improvements that were statistically significant. (This study had no control group for comparison.)

In another study administered by Michael Young, L.Ac., a practitioner trained at Quan Yin, of 150 patients who completed a twelve-week uncontrolled trial, many reported reduction of chronic HIV-related complaints and improvement in quality of life. According to Misha Cohen, L.Ac., OMD, and other practitioners, laboratory changes are often not as dramatic as symptomatic ones.

The San Francisco General Hospital Study

This study was undertaken in early 1993. The principal investigators were Jeff Burack, M.D., of San Francisco General Hospital and Misha Cohen, L.Ac., OMD, of Quan Yin Healing Arts Center. The herbs used in the study were donated by Health Concerns, and the placebo was funded by the University of California at San Francisco.

The objectives of the study were to evaluate the safety, efficacy, and toxicity of a preparation of Chinese herbs while attempting to reduce the patients' symptoms and improve their well-being. Subjects chosen had moderately advanced, symptomatic HIV infection. Thirty subjects were enrolled by January 1993. Twenty-eight (93%) were male; 19 (63%) were white; 4 (13%) Latino; 4 (13%) African-American; and 3 (10%) other. Median age was 36 years (range: 26-59). Median baseline CD4 count was 303 (range: 210-408). Fifteen were taking nucleoside analog anti-retrovirals prior to and during the study.

A randomized, double-blind, placebo-controlled, twelve-week pilot study was conducted. Subjects were HIV-infected adults with CD4 counts of 200-500, without an AIDS diagnosis, and experiencing at least two HIV-related symptoms. Subjects took 28 pills per day of either a standardized preparation of Chinese herbs selected for their antiviral and immunomodulatory properties, or an identical placebo. Chief outcome variables were changes from baseline in overall well-being, physical and social functioning, and symptoms. Secondary outcome variables included changes in weight, CD4 count, hemoglobin, depression, anxiety, and adherence to regimens.

Fifteen participants received a Chinese herbal preparation, and fifteen received an herbal placebo. The herbal preparation was a combination of Enhance and Clear Heat, which have been used extensively in treating HIV infection. The placebo tablet was composed of microcrystalline cellulose. The administration of the herbs (and placebo) was seven tablets QID on an empty stomach. The total herb substance (including extracts) was 18.2 grams per day. Median compliance was 28 tablets per day.

Preliminary results indicate that life satisfaction improved significantly in the Chinese formula group as compared to the placebo group (median test p=.02). Improvement was also observed in fatigue (p=.046), gastrointestinal (p=.02), and neurological symptoms (p=.04) in the herb group versus the placebo group. Moderate improvement in pain (p=.136) and sleep (p=.058) were also seen. Other symptoms tested, as well as CD4 counts and other laboratory parameters, did not exhibit any statistically significant changes. Interestingly, dermatological symptoms improved in the placebo group, perhaps due to anomaly or to the increase in fiber consumed. One patient who received the placebo developed diarrhea which required discontinuation of the study. Otherwise, none of the remaining subjects in either group experienced toxicity symptoms.

While the results of this and other studies are important, research with larger numbers of subjects and undertaken over longer periods should be conducted in order to confirm the present findings. We hope that a private source of funding will help continue this valuable research.

Herbal Formulas Used in Treating HIV

When treating HIV patients, base formulas are used with adjunct ones. Quan Yin primarily uses tablets that have been specifically developed for HIV patients. An advantage of such forms of administration is high patient compliance which allows for attainment of a higher overall dosage than that for decoctions. Most patients do not have the time, living arrangements, or money to brew decoctions on a continual basis. A number of formulas have been used in the past at Quan Yin to treat HIV patients, including Astra 8, Ganoderma 18, Power Mushrooms, and Composition A. The present formula that is used is Enhance, which was developed by Misha Cohen based on the clinical experience at Quan Yin. Enhance was designed to be easily digested and assimilated. The adjunct formulas used are Clear Heat and Marrow Plus.

TCM Approach to HIV Treatment

According to Misha Cohen, the Spleen and Stomach are the first Organs attacked by the HIV virus. The results are a weakened digestive and diminished Spleen/Stomach function. Lifestyle factors contribute to injury of Kidney energy and other systems such as the Lung. AIDS-diagnosed patients typically have the above deficiencies along with deficiency-Heat, Blood stagnation, and Shen disturbances. The terminal stage of AIDS is characterized by exhaustion or collapse of Qi and Blood in all the Organs. Therefore, when treating HIV patients, remedies should be aimed at supporting the Organs, in addition to addressing other pathologic factors.

Most HIV-infected patients present minute red spots on the tongue. Occasionally these are difficult to see, and at other times they are very red and visible. Such spots are an indication of Toxic Heat, as are inflammatory responses like pruritus, sore throat, elevated body temperature, and feverish sensation.

In terms of treatment, the strategy is to clear Heat and relieve Toxicity. Herbs with these capabilities have been found through laboratory and clinical research to possess anti-viral properties. Formulas such as Clear Heat and Enhance contain such herbs; however, the former is made up solely of these herbs and thus should not be administered alone for long periods. Enhance, on the other hand, contains additional herbs that protect the Spleen/Stomach. Clear Heat also possesses Laminaria (Kun Bu) which addresses lymph node swelling, a common symptom in HIV infection.

Some patients, after starting on herbal formulas, suffer digestive difficulties such as diarrhea and/or constipation. This is usually due to the increase in fiber. Therefore, it is advisable that patients use half the normal dose during the first few days. They can also experiment with taking the formulas with or after meals, although the latter is not recommended since herbs are absorbed more rapidly on an empty stomach. Patients may discover that herbs are easier to absorb during certain times of the day. For example, some individuals have difficulty digesting herbs in the morning, but not in the afternoon. If these strategies are unsuccessful, then Quiet Digestion can be added to the regimen.

Most American practitioners are now combining TCM and Western modalities in treating HIV infection. In fact, Chinese herbs can actually help HIV patients better tolerate some pharmaceuticals by reducing or even eliminating their side effects. For example, Marrow Plus which contains Blood-tonifying and Blood-vitalizing herbs (traditionally aimed at strengthening the bone marrow) was developed specifically to counter anemia and other side effects of AZT and chemotherapy. Currently, we are testing a formula that addresses chronic watery stools in HIV-infected patients diagnosed with cryptosporidium. As always, it is recommended that patients use herbs under the supervision of an experienced practitioner. Practitioners with a special interest in treating HIV/AIDS may attend a certificate training course offered by Quan Yin Healing Arts Center.

Appendix D
Antiviral Properties of Clear Heat

Andrew Gaeddert, TCM Herbalist
Nissi S. Wang, M.Sc.

One of the more promising areas of Chinese herbal research is on herbs that possess antiviral properties. The Health Concerns' formula Clear Heat, which was developed by Misha Cohen, OMD, L.Ac., at Quan Yin Clinic, is for the treatment of viral conditions. It is usually used in combination with Enhance or Astra Isatis for HIV infection, chronic fatigue immune dysfunction syndrome (CFIDS), or herpes infection. Enhance and Astra Isatis also contain antiviral herbs, although the primary action of these two formulas is tonification. Clear Heat has also been used successfully with Isatis Gold in treating Lyme disease, and with Ecliptex for hepatitis.The herbs in Clear Heat were selected for their antiviral, antibacterial, and antifungal properties. This article presents the antiviral properties of the herbs in this formula.

The chief herb in Clear Heat is Isatis extract which is derived from *Isatis tinctoria*, and is composed of Ban Lan Gen (the root of Isatis) and Da Qing Ye (the leaf). Much research has been conducted in China on the antiviral effects of Ban Lan Gen and Da Qing Ye. *In vitro* studies found extracts of Ban Lan Gen to have an inhibitory action against certain influenza strains, and Da Qing Ye against the encephalitis B and mumps viruses, as well as against influenza. Clinical studies show good results for Ban Lan Gen and Da Qing Ye in treating encephalitis B, chickenpox, hepatitis, mumps, influenza, infectious mononucleosis, viral skin diseases, and other viral conditions.

In forty-three cases of infectious mononucleosis treated with intramuscular injection of Ban Lan Gen and oral administration of its decoction, rapid improvement in subjective symptoms, rapid lowering of body temperature and decrease of abnormal lymphocytes were noted; cure was achieved in three to five days, with young children responding better than adults.

Although Ban Lan Gen and Da Qing Ye have not yet been found to be virucidal against HIV in laboratory studies, their traditional use is for conditions of Heat due to Toxin in the Blood, which may make these two herbs appropriate for treating persons with HIV.

Lonicera (Jin Yin Hua) is another herb in the formula which clears Heat and expels Toxin. It has a broad antibacterial effect against micro-organisms such as *Staphylococcus aureus*, *Streptococcus hemolyticus*, *Shigella dysenteriae*,and *Salmonella*, among others. Clinically, in addition to addressing conditions caused by the aforementioned bacteria, Lonicera has been used for treating viral diseases such as infectious hepatitis and upper respiratory infections due to influenza.

The traditional effects of Prunella (Xia Ku Cao) are to clear Liver Heat and disperse masses especially due to Phlegm Fire. Laboratory studies have found decoctions of Prunella to be inhibitory against various bacteria. The herb has been used to treat tuberculosis of the lymph nodes, acute icteric hepatitis, and hypertension. An important study by Chang and Yeung in 1988 found Prunella to cause direct inhibition of the growth of HIV *in vitro*.

Chang and Yeung also found Andrographis (Chuan Xin Lian) to inhibit HIV. Because of its Heat-clearing and Toxin-expelling effects, Andrographis treats infectious conditions such as bacillary dysentery, respiratory infections, otitis media, among other diseases. Many laboratory and clinical studies have been conducted on its antiviral actions against diseases such as herpes zoster, chicken pox, mumps, and hepatitis.

Of the twenty-seven herbs tested by Chang and Yeung, Viola (Zi Hua Di Ding) possessed the strongest inhibitory effect against HIV *in vitro*. Viola's traditional effects are clearing Heat and eliminating Toxin, and relieving inflammation. Classical formulas that treat carbuncles, deep-rooted furuncles, and malignant lesions often have Viola as one of their main ingredients. Viral infections such as mumps may be treated with Viola as well.

The remaining herbs in Clear Heat — Oldenlandia (Bai Hua She She Cao), Cordyceps (Dong Chong Xia Cao), and Licorice (Gan Cao) — also possess antibacterial, antiviral, and antifungal effects, but to lesser degrees than the other herbs. For example, Cordyceps has been found to inhibit the growth of various bacteria such as *Staphylococcus*, *Streptococcus*, *Bacillus anthracis*, and *Mycobacterium avium*, among others. Extensive studies have been conducted on Licorice; in addition to its actions on the endocrine system and its ability to treat gastric and duodenal ulcers, it is used clinically to treat infectious hepatitis, inflammatory diseases of the eye such as herpetic keratitis, and other infectious conditions. In Clear Heat, Licorice not only serves as an added antibacterial and antiviral herb, but also harmonizes the other ingredients and guides them to enter their respective channels.

The aforementioned antiviral herbs are mostly cool in property and address symptoms of Heat. Experience among American practitioners shows that although patients with viral conditions may present with Cold signs, they can still benefit from antiviral herbs because the virus is most likely latent and should be attacked. In these cases and in individuals who will receive antiviral herbs for longer than two to three weeks, tonifying formulas/herbs should also be given in order to protect the digestive system from injury due to long-term use of cooling herbs.

The following case histories of patients at Quan Yin Clinic in San Francisco illustrate the clinical use of Clear Heat.

Case Studies

Case 1

This patient is a thirty-nine year-old white woman who was seen by Abigail Surasky, L.Ac. The patient had symptoms of premenstrual syndrome (PMS), including breast distention, bouts of anger, irritability, depression, cravings, hot flashes, night sweats, and restlessness. She had also received a biomedical diagnosis of chronic fatigue immune dysfunction syndrome (CFIDS), the symptoms of which are extreme fatigue, panic, muscle aches, joint pain, and fevers. Her digestion was generally fine.

After one month of six acupuncture treatments, and in spite of possible complications of receiving a flu injection prior to the sixth treatment, her PMS symptoms diminished, her emotional outlook improved, her energy was somewhat restored. Her energy remained low, however, and she was still slightly feverish. Following the sixth treatment she moved away from San Francisco and discontinued acupuncture. During her final session she was given Clear Heat to take along. One month later she called to indicate that her energy was much improved and the Heat symptoms had all but disappeared. She attributed her improved health to taking Clear Heat.

Case 2

This patient is a twenty-seven year-old white man who was seen by Misha Cohen, OMD, L.Ac. The patient had persistent anal warts which resisted treatment with liquid nitrogen, podophyllin, laser surgery, and electrocauterization during a five month period; the condition returned two to three weeks following each treatment. His first two sessions at Quan Yin involved only acupuncture. At the third session he was asked to take Clear Heat. Four weeks later, the patient reported that the warts were much less intense. At this time, he decided to undergo Efudex treatment (chemotherapy) because he was leaving the country soon. The warts disappeared completely following Efudex. The patient took several bottles of Clear Heat with him on his trip. One year later he returned to the U.S. and indicated that the Clear Heat had maintained the warts at a very low level of activity. He believed that the combined drug and herbal approach had been his best course.

Case 3
This is a fifty-five year-old woman who was also seen by Misha Cohen. The patient had a biomedical diagnosis of CFIDS, and more recently, Crohn's disease. She had been receiving acupuncture and herbal treatments since 1983 with excellent results. The CFIDS is controlled with various herbal formulas and weekly acupuncture; initially, she had required two acupuncture treatments per week. She had not been taking herbs for the CFIDS for several months, and had recently experienced a recurrence of viral symptoms such as hot flashes, sore throat, fatigue, and body aches. She presented with a rapid thready pulse, and a tongue with little coating and a red center. She was advised to begin a course of Clear Heat, and within one week she reported increased energy and fewer bouts of sore throats and hot flashes. After six weeks she claimed greatly increased energy and no sore throats or sensations of heat. She continues on the Clear Heat because her pulse remains rapid and the tongue red, although less so.

Appendix E
Supplementary Formulas

Many formulas not listed in this section appear in chapters through-out the book. See the index of formulas on page 218 or the general index on page 221 to find formulas not listed here.

Adrenosen
Wild Yam Herbal System

Ingredients

English	pinyin
Wild Yam root	Dioscorea villosa
L-Phenylalanine	
Inosine	Hypoxanthine riboside
PAK	Pyridoxal alpha Ketoglutarate
Prince Ginseng	Tai Zi Shen
Dioscorea	Shan Yao
Dolichos	Bian Dou
Schizandra	Wu Wei Zi
Oryza	Gu Ya
Chinese malt	Mai Ya

Antler 8

Ingredients

English	pinyin
Deer antler	Lu rong
Salvia	Dan Shen
Dendrobium	Shi Hu
Rehmannia (raw)	Sheng Di Huang
Tortoise shell	Gui Ban
Tang-kuei	Dang Gui
Aquilaria	Chen Xiang
Cardamon	Sha Ren

Aquilaria 22

Ingredients

English	*pinyin*
Aquilaria	Chen Xiang
Ginger	Gan Jiang
Mume	Wu Mei
Codonopsis	Dang Shen
Myrobalan	He Zi
Poria	Fu Ling
Atractylodes	Bai Zhu
Quisqualis	Shi Jun Zi
Omphalia	Lei Wan
Saussurea	Mu Xiang
Torreya	Fei Zi
Pomegranate	Shi Liu Pi
Melia	Chuan Lian Zi
Rubia	Fu Pen Zi
Chi-Shih	Zhi Shi
Nutmeg	Rou Dou Kou
Cardamon	Bai Dou Kou
Ulmus	Wu Yi
Zanthoxylum	Hua Jiao
Licorice	Gan Cao
Aloe Vera	Lu Hui

Arouse Vigor

Ingredients

English	*pinyin*
Astragalus	Huang Qi
Ginseng	Ren Shen
Tang-kuei	Dang Gui
Baked licorice	Zhi Gan Cao
Tangerine peel	Chen Pi
Cimicifuga	Sheng Ma
Bupleurum	Chai Hu
Atractylodes	Bai Zhu

Aspiration
Polygala Far Reaching Formula

Ingredients

English	Latin/*pinyin*
Polygala	Yuan Zhi
Vervain	Herba Verbenae Officinalis
Gambir	Gou Teng
Gardenia	Zhi Zi
Albizzia flowers	He Huan Hua
Damiana	Folium Turnerae Aphrodisiaciae
White Peony	Bai Shao
Tang-kuei	Dang Gui
Pinellia	Ban Xia
Poria	Fu Ling
Aquilaria	Chen Xiang

Astra 8
Astragalus 8 Combination

Ingredients

English	*pinyin*
Astragalus	Huang Qi
Ligustrum	Nu Zhen Zi
Ganoderma	Ling Zhi
Eleutheroginseng	Ci Wu Jia
Codonopsis	Dang Shen
Schizandra	Wu Wei Zi
Licorice	Gan Cao
Oryza	Gu Ya
Malt	Mai Ya

Astra Diet Tea
Caffeine Free

Ingredients

English	*pinyin*
Peppermint	Bo He
Eleutheroginseng	Ci Wu Jia
Ginger	Gan Jiang
Loquat	Pi Pa Ye
Perilla leaf	Zi Su Ye
Lophatherum leaf	Dan Zhu Ye

Bioradiance

Ingredients

Gentiana campestris

Sanguinaria canadensis

Impatiens pallida

Hydrastis canadensis

Ferula galbaniflua

Fumaria officinalis

Frasera carolinensis

Allicin

Chlorophyllin

trace elements

Celosia 10

Ingredients

English	pinyin
Celosia	Qing Xiang Zi
Rehmannia, raw	Sheng Di Huang
Salvia	Dan Shen
Red Peony	Chi Shao
Eclipta	Han Lian Cao
San chi	San Qi
Sophora flower	Huai Hua
Chrysanthemum	Ju Hua
Lycium fruit	Gou Qi Zi
Tang-kuei	Dang Gui

Clear Air
Ma-Huang and Tussilago Formula

Ingredients

English	pinyin
Ma-huang Concentrate	Ma Huang
Tussilago Concentrate	Kuan Dong Hua
Perilla Fruit	Su Zi
Apricot Seed	Ku Xing Ren
Morus Bark	Sang Bai Pi
Tricosanthes Root	Tian Hua Fen
Fritillaria	Zhe Bei Mu
Aristolachia	Ma Dou Ling
Aster	Zi Wan
Belamcanda	She Gan
Scute	Huang Qin
Schizandra	Wu Wei Zi
Licorice	Gan Cao
Pinellia	Ban Xia

Clearing
Modified Heart-Clearing Lotus Seed Tablets

Ingredients

English	pinyin
Lotus Seed	Lian Zi
Ophiopogon	Mai Men Dong
Poria	Fu Ling
White Ginseng	Jilin Ren Shen
Plantaginis	Che Qian Zi
Scutellaria	Huang Qin
Comfrey Root	Gan Fu Li
Smilax	Tu Fu Ling
Astragalus	Huang Qi
Lycium Bark	Di Gu Pi
Moutan	Mu Dan Pi
Red Peony	Chi Shao
Licorice	Gan Cao

Colorful Phoenix Pearl Combo

Ingredients

English	pinyin
Pearl	Zhen Zhu
Mother of Pearl	Zhen Zhu Mu
Rehmannia	Shu Di Huang
Adenophora	Nan Sha Shen
Scrophularia	Xuan Shen
Lonicera	Jin Yin Hua
Phellodendron	Huang Bai
Rhubarb	Da Huang

Ease Plus
Bupleurum Plus Combination

Ingredients

English	pinyin
Oystershell calcium	Mu Li & Long Gu
Bupleurum	Chai Hu
Ginseng	Ren Shen
Ginger	Gan Jiang
Pinellia	Ban Xia
Scute	Huang Qin
Cinnamon	Gui Zhi
Rhubarb	Da Huang
Saussurea	Mu Xiang

Eight Treasures
Tang Kuei and Ginseng Eight Herbal Formula
Ba Zhen Tang

Ingredients

English	pinyin
Codonopsis	Dang Shen
Atractylodes	Bai Zhu
Poria	Fu Ling
Rehmannia	Shu Di Huang
Peony	Bai Shao
Tang Kuei	Dang Gui
Ligusticum	Chuan Xiong
Milletia	Ji Xue Teng
Baked Licorice	Zhi Gan Cao
Ginger	Gan Jiang
Red Dates	Da Zao

Eupolyphaga Tablets

Ingredients

English	*pinyin*
Eupolyphaga	Zhe Chong
Rhubarb	Da Huang
Rehmannia, raw	Sheng Di Huang
Peony	Bai Shao
Earthworm	Di Long
Leech	Shui Zhi
Tabanus	Meng Chong
Holotrichia	Qi Cao
Persica	Tao Ren
Scute	Huang Qin
Licorice	Gan Cao
Lacca	Gan Qi

Gather Vitality

Ingredients

English	*pinyin*
Ginseng	Ren Shen
Astragalus	Huang Qi
Atractylodes	Bai Zhu
Poria	Fu Ling
Zizyphus	Suan Zao Ren
Longan	Long Yan Rou
Saussurea	Mu Xiang
Baked licorice	Zhi Gan Cao
Tang-kuei	Dang Gui
Polygala	Yuan Zhi
Ginger	Gan Jiang
Red Dates	Da Zao

Heavenly Water
Gotu Kola 15 Formula

Ingredients

English	Latin/*pinyin*
Gotu Kola	Hydrocotyle asiatica
Chaste Tree Berries	Viticis Agnus-casti
Passion Flower	Passiflorae Incarnatae
Pseudostellaria	Tai Zi Shen
Scute	Huang Qin
Pinellia	Ban Xia
Poria	Fu Ling
Peony	Bai Shao
Tang-kuei	Dang Gui
Cyperus	Xiang Fu
Tricosanthes	Gua Lou Ren
Red Dates	Da Zao
Baked Licorice	Zhi Gan Cao
Citrus	Chen Pi
Blue Citrus	Qing Pi

Lithospermum 15

Ingredients

English	*pinyin*
Lithospermum	Zi Cao
Salvia	Dan Shen
Astragalus	Huang Qi
Smilax	Tu Fu Ling
Red peony	Chi Shao
Cistanche	Rou Cong Rong
Rehmannia	Shou Di Huang
Ligustrum	Niu Zhen Zi
Epimedium	Yin Yang Huo
Codonopsis	Dang Shen
Artemesia anua	Qing Hao
Anemarrhena	Zhi Mu
Lycium fruit	Gou Qi Zi
Tang-kuei	Dang Gui
Licorice	Gan Cao

Lucid Channel

Ingredients

English	pinyin
Citrus	Chen Pi
Pinellia	Ban Xia
Poria	Fu Ling
Baked licorice	Zhi Gan Cao
Bitter Orange	Zhi Shi
Jack-in-the-Pulpit	Tian Nan Xing
Acorus	Shi Chang Pu

Meridian Circulation

Ingredients

English	pinyin
Du Huo	Du Huo
Qin Jiao	Qin Jiao
Siler	Fang Feng
Mulberry mistletoe	Sang Ji Sheng
Eucommia	Du Zhong
Cyathula	Chuan Niu Xi
Cinnamon bark	Rou Gui
Tang kuei	Dang Gui
Peony	Bai Shao
Ginseng	Ren Shen
Baked licorice	Zhi Gan Cao
Poria	Fu Ling
Coral bean bark	Hai Tong Pi
Aristolochia	Guang Fang Ji
Cibot	Gou Ji

Minor Blue Dragon
Herbal Concentrate

Ingredients

English	pinyin
Pinellia	Ban Xia
Licorice	Gan Cao
Schizandra	Wu Wei Zi
Ma-huang	Ma Huang
Cinnamon	Gui Zhi
Ginger	Gan Jiang
Peony	Bai Shao
Asarum	Xi Xin

Prosperous Farmer

Ingredients

English	pinyin
Ginseng	Ren Shen
Atractylodes	Bai Zhu
Poria	Fu Ling
Astragalus	Huang Qi
Licorice	Gan Cao
Dioscorea	Shan Yao
Ginger	Gan Jiang
Citrus	Chen Pi
Pinellia	Ban Xia
Amomum	Sha Ren
Saussurea	Mu Xiang
Magnolia	Hou Po
Crataegus	Shan Zha

Rehmannia 8
Herbal Concentrate

Ingredients

English	*pinyin*
Rehmannia	Shu Di Huang
Poria	FuLing
Moutan	MuDanPi
Dioscorea	ShanYao
Cornus	Shan Zhu Yu
Alisma	Ze Xie
Eucommia	Du Zhong
Cinnamon Bark	Rou Gui

Shen-Gem

Ingredients

English	*pinyin*
Ginseng	Ren Shen
Poria	Fu Ling
White Atractylodes	Bai Zhu
Zizyphus	Suan Zao Ren
Astragalus	Huang Qi
Tang-kuei	Dang Gui
Salvia	Dan Shen
Amber	Hu Po
Polygala	Yuan Zhi
Longan	Long Yan Rou
Saussurea	Mu Xiang
Ginger	Gan Jiang
Licorice	Gan Cao
Cardamon	Sha Ren

Source Qi

Ingredients

English	pinyin
Astragalus	Huang Qi
Ginseng	Ren Shen
White Atractylodes	Bai Zhu
Poria	Bai Fu Ling
Dioscorea	Shan Yao
Lotus seed	Lian Rou
Euryales	Qian Shi
Cimicifuga	Sheng Ma
Bupluerum	Chai Hu
Ginger	Gan Jiang
Nutmeg seeds	Rou Dou Kou
Baked Licorice	Zhi Gan Cao
Ailanthus	Chun Bai Pi

SPZM

Ingredients

English	pinyin
Peony	Bai Shao
Pueraria	Ge Gen
Clematis	Wei Ling Xian
Milletia	Ji Xue Teng
Licorice	Gan Cao
Calcium Aspartate	
Magnesium Aspartate	

Temper Fire

Ingredients

English	*pinyin*
Rehmannia	Shu Di Huang
Cornus	Shan Zhu Yu
Dioscorea	Shan Yao
Alisma	Ze Xie
Moutan	Mu Dan Pi
Poria	Fu Ling
Anemarrhena	Zhi Mu
Phellodendron	Huang Bai

Wise Judge

Ingredients

English	*pinyin*
Glehnia	Sha Shen
Ophiopogon	Mai Men Dong
Yu Zhu	Yu Zhu
Asparagus	Tian Men Dong
Lily	Bai He
Platycodon	Jie Geng
Fritallaria	Zhe Bei Mu
Tang Kuei	Dang Gui
Rehmannia	Shu Di Huang
Tremella	Bai Mu Er
American Ginseng	Xi Yang Shen
Licorice	Gan Cao
Poria	Fu Ling
Prince Ginseng	Tai Zi Shen
Schizandra	Wu Wei Zi

Yin Chao Jin

Ingredients

English	*pinyin*
Lonicera	Jin Yin Hua
Forsythia	Lian Qiao
Isatis Extract	Ban Lan Gen &
	Da Qing Ye
Arctium	Niu Bang Zi
Mentha	Bo He
Schizonepeta	Jing Jie
Soja	Dan Dou Chi
Platycodon	Jie Geng
Lophaterum	Dan Zhu Ye
Phragmites	Lu Gen
Licorice	Gan Cao

Zedoaria Tablets

Ingredients

English	*pinyin*
Zedoaria	E Zhu
Oldenlandia	Bai Hua She She Cao
Gleditsia spine	Zao Ci
Sparganium	San Leng
Curcuma	Yu Jin
Acorus	Chuan Pu
Frankincense	Ru Xiang
Euployphaga	Zhe Chong

Bibliography

Anon. *A Barefoot Doctor's Manual*. Philadelphia: Running Press, 1977.

Balch, James F. and Phyllis A. Balch. *Prescription for Nutritional Healing*. Garden City Park, NY: Avery Publishing Group, Inc, 1990.

Beinfield, Harriet and Efrem Korngold. *Between Heaven and Earth*. New York: Ballantine, 1991.

Bensky, Dan and Andrew Gamble. *Chinese Herbal Medicine Materia Medica*. Revised edition. Seattle: Eastland Press, 1986.

Bensky, Dan and Randall Barolet. *Chinese Herbal Medicine Formulas and Strategies*. Seattle: Eastland Press, 1990.

Chang, Hson-Mou and Paul Pui-Hay But, ed. *Pharmacology and Applications of Chinese Materia Medica*. Vols 1 and 2. Singapore: World Scientific Publishing Co, 1986.

Chen, Ze-lin and Mei-fang Chen. *A Comprehensive Guide to Chinese Herbal Medicine*. Long Beach, CA: Oriental Healing Arts Institute, 1992.

Dharmananda, Subhuti. *Chinese Herbal Therapies for Immune Disorders*. Portland, OR: Institute for Traditional Medicine, 1988.

——— . *From the Peoples's Pharmacy*. Portland, OR: Institute for Traditional Medicine, 1989.

——— . *Prescriptions on Silk and Paper*. Portland, OR: Institute for Traditional Medicine, 1989.

——— . *A Bag of Pearls*. Portland, OR: Institute for Traditional Medicine, revised 1993.

Enquin, Zhang, ed. *Clinic of Traditional Chinese Medicine*. Vols 1 and 2. China: Shanghai College of Traditional Chinese Medicine, 1990.

——— . *Prescriptions of Traditional Chinese Medicine*. China: Shanghai College of Traditional Chinese Medicine, 1990.

Flaws, Bob. *Arisal of the Clear*. Boulder, CO: Blue Poppy Press, 1991.

Fratkin, Jake Paul. *Chinese Classics*. Santa Fe, NM: Shya Publications, 1990.

Gaeddert, Andrew. *Health Concerns Clinical Manual*. Alameda, CA: Health Concerns, 1990.

Gong, Xiao and Zuo Lian-jun. *The Treatment of Knotty Diseases*. Jinan, China: Shandong Science and Technology Press, 1990.

Hammer, Leon. *Dragon Rises, Red Bird Flies*. Barrytown, NY: Station Hill Press, 1990.

Hsu, Hong-yen and Chau-shin Hsu. *Commonly Used Chinese Herb Formulas with Illustrations*. Long Beach, CA: Oriental Healing Arts Institute, 1980.

Hsu, Hong-yen, and Yuh-pan Chen, Shuenn-jyi Shen, Chau-shin Hsu, Chien-chih Chen, Hsien-chang Chang. *Oriental Materia Medica*. Long Beach, CA: Oriental Healing Arts Institute, 1986.

Kaptchuk, Ted J. *The Web That Has No Weaver*. Chicago: Congdon & Weed, 1983.

——— . *K'an Herbals Formula Guide*. Revised ed. Aptos, CA: Sanders Enterprises, 1992.

Kohn, Livia, ed. *Taoist Meditation and Longevity Techniques*. Ann Arbor, MI: University of Michigan, 1989.

Maciocia, Giovanni. *The Foundations of Chinese Medicine*. Edinburgh: Churchill Livingstone, 1989.

Marcus, Alon. *Acute Abdominal Syndromes*. Boulder, CO: Blue Poppy Press, 1991.

Margolis, Simeon and Hamilton Moses III, ed. *The Johns Hopkins Medical Handbook*. New York: Rebus, Inc, 1992.

Murray, Michael and Joseph Pizzorno. *Encyclopedia of Natural Medicine*. Rocklin, CA: Prima Publishing, 1991.

Naeser, Margaret A. *Outline Guide to Chinese Herbal Patent Medicines in Pill Form.* Boston, MA: Boston Chinese Medicine, 1990.

O'Connor, John and Dan Bensky, ed. *Acupuncture: A Comprehensive Text.* Seattle, WA: Eastland Press, 1981.

Unschuld, Paul U. *Forgotten Traditions of Ancient Chinese Medicine.* Brookline, MA: Paradigm Publications, 1990.

Xuezhong, Shuai. *Fundamentals of Traditional Chinese Medicine.* Beijing, China: Foreign Languages Press, 1992.

Yanchi, Liu. *The Essential Book of Traditional Chinese Medicine*, Vol 2. New York: Columbia University Press, 1988.

Yeung, Him-che. *Handbook of Chinese Herbs and Formulas.* Vols 1 and 2. Los Angeles: Institute of Chinese Medicine, 1985.

Zhang, Qingcai and Hong-yen Hsu. *AIDS and Chinese Medicine.* Long Beach, CA: Oriental Healing Arts Institute, 1990.

Zhu, Chun-Han. *Clinical Handbook of Chinese Prepared Formulas.* Brookline, MA: Paradigm Publications, 1989.

Zhufan, Xie and Huang Xiakai, ed. *Dictionary of Traditional Chinese Medicine.* Hong Kong: The Commercial Press, Ltd, 1984.

Glossary of Terms

Blood

Blood is the most dense fluid in the body. The Chinese concept of Blood also includes the subtle matrix that contains the mental and emotional life.

Blood Stagnation, Blood Stasis

A condition where Blood moves slowly, congeals, or forms clots. This includes bruises and some other painful conditions such as some menstrual irregularities. Blood Stagnation can be due to Cold, Heat, deficiency, or trauma.

Burner (Jiao)

The upper burner is the area of the body above the diaphragm, and includes the heart, lungs, and head. The middle burner, which relates to digestion, lies between the navel and the diaphragm and includes the stomach, spleen, liver, and gallbladder. The lower burner is the area below the navel, and includes the kidneys and bladder, intestines, reproductive organs, and the liver and gallbladder channels.

Cold

A condition of reduced metabolic activity, characterized by feelings of cold or sleepiness.

Damp

Watery accumulations in organs or cavities as a result of weakness of the Spleen. This may be accompanied by feelings of heaviness, swelling, abdominal distension, phlegmatic discharges, nodular masses, or watery stool.

Damp Heat

A combination of excess Damp and excess Heat, usually affecting the Spleen or digestive organs and accompanied by excess Phlegm.

Deficiency

A condition of reduced function or diminished capacity of an organ or process. The Chinese concept of Deficiency also includes decreased resistance to stress or infection.

Deficiency Heat

A condition of Heat signs that are due to a deficiency of the *Yin*. Therapy for Deficiency Heat usually includes nourishing the *Yin* as well as clearing the Heat.

Essence (Jing)

"Jing" is usually translated as Essence. It is the subtle substance that underlies all organic matter and is the source of organic change. It is the basis for reproduction and development of the organism. Jing irregularities are associated with congenital disorders, and jing naturally becomes deficient in old age.

Excess

A condition of heightened function or obstruction or organ or process. This Chinese concept also includes increased reactivity to stress or infection.

Gallbladder

The Chinese concept of gallbladder includes the physical gallbladder as well as the function of decision-making.

Heat

Elevated metabolic activity, inflammation, characterized by sensations of heat or warmth.

Heart

The Chinese concept of Heart includes the physical heart as well as the arterial system, the complexion, the tongue, the external ear, and the functions of awareness in the conscious mind, propulsion of Blood, and containment of the Shen, or spirit.

Kidney

The Chinese concept of Kidney includes the physical kidney as well as the adrenal glands, ovaries, testes, brain, spinal column, bones, teeth, anus, urethra, and inner ear, as well as the functions of fluid balance, reproduction, and growth.

Large Intestine

The Chinese concept of Large Intestine includes the physical large intestine as well as the processes of elimination of solid wastes and psychological release.

Liver

The Chinese concept of Liver includes the physical liver as well as the tendons, ligaments, external genitalia, and the functions of storing Blood and regulating the flow of Blood, Qi, and emotions.

Liver Fire

Fever in the liver that rises towards the head, with symptoms that can include headache, nausea, burning eyes, conjunctivitis, ringing in the ears, and insomnia.

Lung

The Chinese concept of Lung includes the physical lung and respiratory apparatus, the skin and hair, and the processes of refining Qi, maintaining rhythm, and upholding boundaries and surface defenses.

Phlegm

Congealed Damp, formed in Damp Heat conditions or Cold conditions. Phlegm may accumulate in the intestines, lungs, uterus, sinuses, or acupuncture channels. Phlegm may be deposited throughout the body as nodules, lumps, or tumors. It may be stored as fatty deposits in the heart and blood vessels.

Pulse

Pulse diagnosis in Traditional Chinese Medicine is much more sophisticated than pulse-taking in Western biomedicine. A TCM practitioner may evaluate the pulse for rate, strength, width, depth, and shape. As many as thirty-two diffeerent pulse patterns are described in classical Chinese texts. Different locations on the wrist also correspond to different TCM organ systems.

Qi

Qi is the vital energy that invigorates and animates the body and its organ functions.

Shen, spirit

The Chinese concept of Shen includes the mind, consciousness, and higher spiritual connection. Disturbed Shen, associated with the Heart, includes mania, disturbing dreams, poor memory, restlessness, and insomnia.

Small Intestine

The Chinese concept of Small Intestine includes the intestinal tract below the Stomach and Liver, and the function of separating out the useful components of food and transmitting wastes to the organs of elimination.

Spleen

The Chinese concept of Spleen includes the physical spleen as well as the pancreas, the lymph network, large muscles, flesh, lips and eyelids, and the functions of extracting and converting nutrients into Blood and Qi.

Spleen Damp

Accumulation of Damp in the Spleen, following deficiency of Spleen Qi. Symptoms may include abdominal distension, loose stools or diarrhea, or indigestion. Spleen Damp may also be the underlying cause of Phlegm in the lungs.

Stomach

The Chinese concept of Stomach includes the physical stomach, and the process of preparation of food to be digested by the Spleen.

Toxin

The Chinese concept of Toxin includes viral or bacterial infection, external pollutants, or accumulated metabolic toxins.

Wind

The Chinese medical concept of Wind includes trembling, twitching, migratory pains, spasm, seizures, itching, and conditions brought on by exposure to the elements.

Yang

The functional aspects of the body and organs, and the generation of metabolic heat. Yang is also translated as "vital function."

Yin

The material aspects of the body, and the functions of cooling and moistening the organs. Yin is also translated as "vital essence."

Table of Formulas

Index

D

E

About the Author

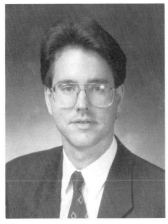

Andrew Gaeddert

Andrew Gaeddert successfully treated himself for Crohn's disease, a gastrointestinal disorder, with Chinese herbal medicine. As a result he founded Health Concerns, a company located in Oakland, California, whose purpose is to spread the benefits of Chinese medicine to millions of Americans suffering form chronic, stress-related, and immune-compromised conditions. In his professional practice, he has helped thousands of people by combining herbal and dietary therapy. For the past ten years, Mr. Gaeddert has studied with master herbalists from both the US and China. In 1992, he assisted in the development of a formula which was the subject of a double-blind clinical trial at University of California San Francisco with HIV patients, the first time an herbal formula has been so carefully evaluated in the U.S. Currently, he is on the protocol team of a study to investigate the effects of Chinese herbs on chronic diarrhea, and an NIH Office of Alternative Medicine funded anemia study.

Mr. Gaeddert is the author of *Chinese Herbs in the Western Clinic* as well as numerous fiction and non-fiction articles. He is also the East Bay coordinator for Citizen for Health, a national non-profit organization that protects health freedom for all Americans.

Mr. Gaeddert, through his inspirational teaching, empowers practitioners and lay people to practice the art of Chinese herbal therapy. He is particularly interested in helping practitioners become successful so they can help Chinese medicine grow.

Practitioners interested sponsoring a seminar in their area, or in tapes, newsletters, or articles by Mr. Gaeddert, may write care of:

Get Well Clinic
8001 Capwell Drive., #A
Oakland, CA 94621

Individuals requesting a referral to a practitioner using herbs may write to the same address.

What practitioners are saying about
Chinese Herbs in the Western Clinic

"I have used similar formulas in my sixty years of practice."

Dr. Fung Fung
author of *Sixty Years in Search of Cures*

"With the increased interest in alternative healing methods, especially herbal therapy, *Chinese Herbs in the Western Clinic* provides practitioners and laypersons with the proper guidance in the use of such remedies. The case histories give invaluable insight into how Chinese medicine is able to resolve conditions that were treated unsuccessfully by conventional medicine.

Nissi Wang, M. Sc.
Author: *Illustrated Dictionary of Chinese Acupuncture,*
            Case Histories From China
            and a forthcoming book on
            traditional Chinese dermatology

"A good general introduction to the use of Chinese herbal medicine. It is especially strong in the areas of viral illness, digestive disorders, and pain syndromes."

Misha Cohen, OMD
Quan Yin Healing Arts Center

Books Available From
Get Well Foundation

Sixty years in Search of Cures

by Dr. Fung Fung $15.95

Sixty Years in Search of Cures is an autobiography of one of the world's most experienced herbalists, Dr. Fung Fung, who routinely saw 100-150 patients per day working in a hospital clinic. This master practitioner, with experience in Canton, Hong Kong, Vietnam, and San Francisco, reveals important dietary and lifestyle habits for the general public and herbal prescriptions for the professional herbalist. (Available May 1994)

Chinese Herbs in the Western Clinic

by Andrew Gaeddert $15.95

Chinese Herbs in the Western Clinic recommends formulas by a variety of manufacturers that have been successfully used with thousands of American patients suffering from immune, digestive, gynecological, respiratory disorders, and other commonly seen complaints such as allergies, anxiety, arthritis, back pain, headaches, injury, insomnia, and stress. Disorders are alphabetized by Western conditions and indexed by traditional Chinese medical terminology for easy reference while patients are in the office. This book is designed for practitioners.

Send check of money order payable to Get Well. Include $2.00 per book shipping and handling. California residents add $1.32 sales tax per book. Please be sure to write your name and address clearly, and to specify the titles and quantities of each book you want. Allow 3 weeks for delivery.

For trade, bookstore, and wholesale inquiries, contact North Atlantic Books, P.O. Box 12327, Berkeley, CA 94701.

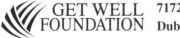 GET WELL FOUNDATION 7172 Regional St. #116
Dublin, CA 94568-2324